Sheffield Hallam University
Learning and IT Services
Adsetts Centre City Campus
Sheffield S1 1WB

AF615194

101 858 159 6

ONE WEEK LOAN

SHEFFIELD HALLAM UNIVERSITY
LEARNING CENTRE
WITHDRAWN FROM STOCK

Tomatoes, Lycopene *and* Human Health

Preventing Chronic Diseases

Edited by Dr. A. Venket Rao

Acknowledgements

The publisher acknowledges with many thanks, the considerable efforts of the Editor in Chief, Venket Rao and of all the authors from around the world who make up the editorial team. Additional thanks also to all at the WPTC and AMITOM, Gwen, Juanjo, Sophie, John, Duncan, Kebede, Ross, Louis, Ed, Tim, David, also Chris Rufer and Cosme. For additional contributions from Juan Jose Amezaga O' Farrell, Diane Barrett, Britt Burton Freeman, Debra Bemis and Gwen Young. Special thanks to all at Lycocard, especially Volker, Angelika and all the consortium. Thank you very much for the attention to the finest of detail in typesetting and sterling design of this book to Jane Darroch Riley with support from Scott, Enzo and Marina and to our editorial department led by Ana Vidal and Jonathan Hawkins and the rest of our team, Amy Thornton, Carine Bouillon, Tarquin, Mike and Diana from Okapi Creative. For silk designs from Jane Sutherland at Alboriginal, Ltr FX from Laura and Cristina. Foundation support team Dorothy and Arthur. Emma et al. This book was brought into being with special support from Ana, Jane D, Zohar, Amy, Rollo and Mrs. Bennet with technical support from Robert and Rebecca Hale, S23. Last minute from Dr. David Jack. Transmission events futures from Oleguer Sarsanedas.

Publisher's Note

The publisher wishes to point out that the manuscripts have been reproduced in the language version in which they were submitted. Therefore some texts are in (BrE) English and others are in (AmE) English. A number of other minor differences in style are visible between the chapters. Again this was to preserve the individual nature of the original texts.

Disclaimer:

The data contained in this publication and any views expressed, belong to the authors and they should not be construed as representing the views of Caledonian Science Press Limited or any distributor of this text

ISBN: 0-9553565-0-4

13-Digit ISBN: 978-0-9553565-0-4

Tomatoes, Lycopene & Human Health, Preventing Chronic Diseases,

Copyright' 2006 by Caledonian Science Press Ltd.

All rights reserved. No part of this publication may be reproduced, stored in a retrieval system or transmitted in any form or by any means, electronically, mechanical, photocopying, recording or otherwise, without the express permission of the publisher. No responsibility is assumed by Tomatoes, Lycopene & Human Health, Preventing Chronic Diseases publisher for any injury and/or damage to persons or property as a result of product liability, negligence or otherwise, or from any use or operation of methods, products, instructions, or ideas contained in the material herein.Because of the rapid advances in the medical sciences, the publisher recommends that independent verification of diagnosis, drug dosages or nutritional advice, should be made.

The Environment:

Caledonian Science press supports a number of different reforestation and tree nursery projects which contribute to sustainable forests. We use the most environmentally friendly materials available to produce our publications and recycle and safely dispose of our waste.

A Catalogue record for this book is available from the British Library.

Printed and Bound in Spain by Gramagraf, C.Corders, Badalona.

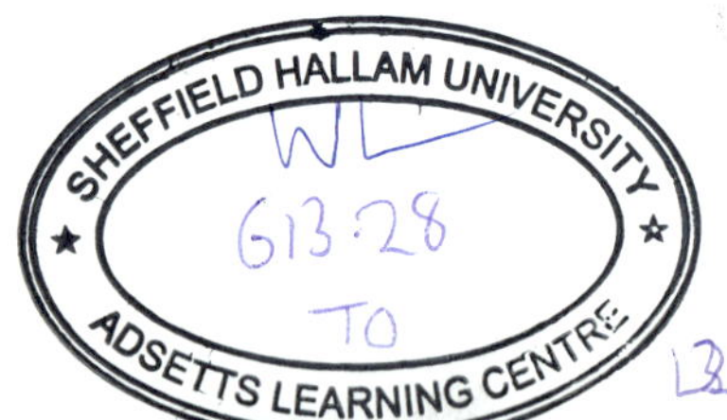

Tomatoes, Lycopene and Human Health

Preventing Chronic Diseases

Edited by Dr. A. Venket Rao

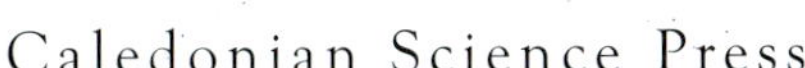

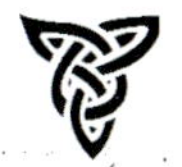

Contents

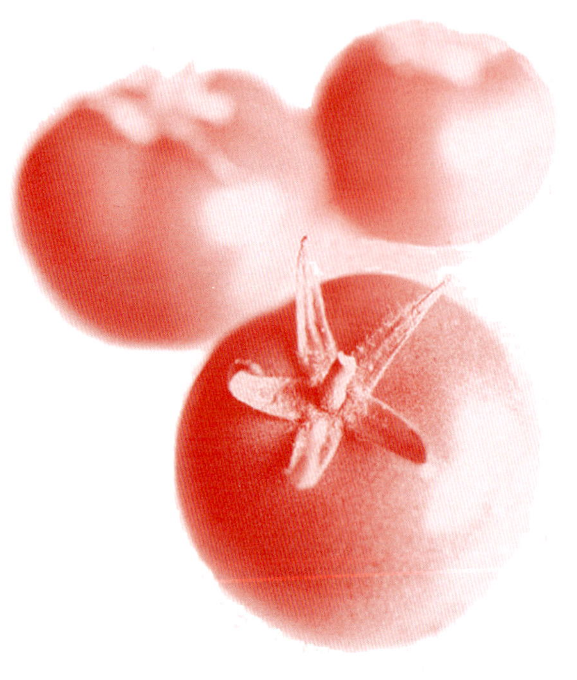

Preface

Dr. Frederick Khachik
University of Maryland

Lycopene and related tomato carotenoids are among the major dietary carotenoids found in human serum, major organs and tissues. During the past decade, numerous *in vitro* and *in vivo* studies have established wide-ranging mechanisms by which lycopene can exert its biological activity in the prevention of chronic diseases in humans.

While the initial focus on research with lycopene began with an epidemiologic study that suggested a protective role of this carotenoid in the prevention of prostate cancer, the health benefits of lycopene in the prevention of other chronic diseases have since been realized.

The contributing authors to this book, who are amongst the World experts on lycopene, have compiled the latest findings from various interdisciplinary research areas to provide the readers with a clear account of the role of this important carotenoid in human health.

The critical evaluation of lycopene in epidemiological and clinical intervention trials as well as details regarding distribution, metabolism, function, and mechanism of action of lycopene, that have been elegantly described in this book, will hopefully stimulate further research with lycopene as well as other dietary carotenoids.

Editorial

Dr. A. Venket Rao
University of Toronto

Scientific evidence strongly supports an association between diet and the prevention of chronic diseases. In recent years there has been a great surge of interest in human health and the role of lycopene, a carotenoid antioxidant present in many fruits and vegetables including tomatoes and tomato products. In the past decade, epidemiological and experimental research activities on lycopene have proliferated exponentially. The *in vitro* properties of lycopene have been well-known for many years. However, a paper published in 1995 suggesting a strong inverse correlation between the consumption of lycopene-containing tomato and tomato products and increased incidence of prostate cancer, initiated the current research activities to evaluate the beneficial role of lycopene beyond prostate cancer to include cancers of other target organs, cardiovascular diseases, diabetes and osteoporosis, among other human diseases. The increasing number of reports on the beneficial potential of lycopene in the prevention of human diseases has led the industries in food, pharmaceutical and cosmeceuticals to take the active and innovative initiative of incorporating lycopene in functional foods. However, the exact mechanisms of action of lycopene are still not understood clearly.

This book was written in response to a need for scientifically sound and state of the art information addressing the role of lycopene in human health. The contributors include a team of scientists, internationally recognized for their expertise in the area of lycopene and human health. The contents of the book cover all aspects of lycopene including its chemistry, analytical methodology, stability, metabolism and its role in chronic diseases including cancer, cardiovascular disease, osteoporosis, male infertility, hypertension and other related human diseases. Recognizing the interest from the industry, chapters have also been included that are authored by experienced and knowledgeable industrial scientists. The contents of this book, therefore, reflect the interests and needs of the scientific community, health professionals, food and related industries and government regulatory agencies.

In view of the increased interest in the role of diet and its components in human health and fast growing functional food and nutraceutical industries, a book such as this is bound to make a significant impact in providing up to date information about lycopene that will help in improving life expectancy and most importantly its quality.

Sincere thanks are extended to all the contributing authors for their excellent coverage of information in their respective areas of expertise. Thanks also to the publisher and the sponsors for their commitment and for making this book a reality.

A. V. Rao
Editor-in-Chief

Foreword

Dr. Ed Giovannucci

Harvard School of Public Health

Lycopene was a relatively ignored compound until about a decade ago, besides some study of its antioxidant properties by a few laboratory scientists. In the past ten years, a number of epidemiologic studies have linked high lycopene intake and blood levels with lower risk of some cancers, particularly prostate cancer, and more recently with reduced risk of cardiovascular diseases.

In addition, interest in lycopene has been generated in regard to other health conditions, including osteoporosis, hypertension, male infertility, and neurodegenerative diseases. Although the epidemiologic studies do not prove a cause and effect association, they have stimulated intense research into potential health benefits of lycopene and lycopene-rich foods, such as tomatoes.

A large and continually increasing number of human dietary intervention studies, animal studies and *in vitro* studies have now been published on various topics related to lycopene. These studies have examined various aspects of lycopene, ranging from basic metabolism and bioavailability, antioxidant properties, to effects on cellular functions, such as how lycopene influences responses to growth factors and affects cell-to-cell communication, and to potential long-term beneficial health effects on populations.

Clearly, lycopene has become of major interest to medical, public health, nutritional, and basic science researchers, as well as to both the food and pharmaceutical industries. Tomatoes, Lycopene and Human Health, edited by Dr. Venket Rao, an international leader in the field, will be a critical book for anyone interested in studying potential uses and benefits of lycopene.

The scope of topics covered is broad and comprehensive, and ranges from the basic chemical properties of lycopene to its potential role in human health at the individual and population level.

Internationally recognized scientists, who are experts in lycopene from various perspectives, author the book's chapters. This book will be an essential reference text and should be useful to anyone interested in this topic, ranging from the novice to the expert.

Dr. Phyllis Bowen

University of Illinois, Chicago.

Carotenoids are a class of compounds that have found great utility in the propagation and maintenance of many life forms. Of the more than 600 carotenoids, lycopene is one of the most intriguing. Its existence in time occurs only in a few plants and only as they mature with the silencing of a single enzyme. Clearly for these plants, its color signals fecundity but does it do more than act as a display and are its properties unique among the many carotenoids? With the discovery of unique risk reduction associations for prostate cancer and then other selected cancers in population studies, there has been a great deal of effort to discover its actions and properties as a single compound and also in the context of the tomato, it's most commonly consumed vehicle. The effort has expanded into exploring risk reduction for other disease processes.

This monograph is indeed timely because it represents the contribution of many researchers and their colleagues toward understanding the properties and bioactivity of lycopene and foods that contain it. Such monographs often serve a foundational function, allowing new researchers to comprehend the scope of the field and sparking new questions, ideas and approaches. Lycopene or its metabolites and oxidation products have clearly shown bioactivity in a number of functional pathways at physiological concentrations. Like many natural compounds, these actions are modest compared to pharmaceuticals developed to block a specific pathway. Yet, if we look at the tomato, with its wealth of secondary bioactive compounds, we see the possibilities of synergy that have been exploited by mother nature, in ways we do not yet understand. As researchers, we shake our heads in chagrin at how we are ever going to sort out the complexities. The effort is well worth it and even becoming tractable. Let us continue.

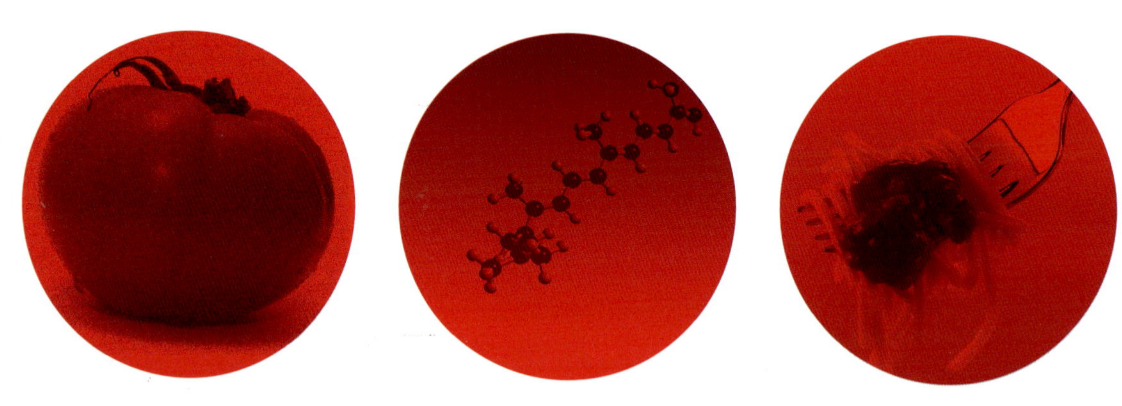

Diet and Chronic Diseases:
Role of Phytonutrients

Dr. A. V. Rao
Department of Nutritional Sciences,
Faculty of Medicine.
University of Toronto,
Ontario, Canada

Abstract

Chronic diseases including cancer, cardiovascular disease, diabetes and osteoporosis are the major causes of morbidity and mortality in the Western World. Along with genetic factors and age, lifestyle factors and diet are also considered important risk factors for these diseases. There is compelling scientific evidence to suggest an important relationship between diet and the incidence of chronic diseases (3,57).

A typical Western diet high in total energy and fat and low in complex carbohydrates including dietary fibre has been causally related to increased risk of cancer and cardiovascular diseases. Based on these observations, dietary guidelines have been formulated around the world for the prevention of chronic diseases. One of the main features of these dietary recommendations is to increase the consumption of plant based foods that include fruits, vegetables, cereals and legumes (2).

A great deal of emphasis has been given in recent years to the consumption of fruits and vegetables for the maintenance of good health and prevention of diseases. Fruits and vegetables mediate their beneficial effects via several mechanisms that include immune modulation, hormonal induction and metabolic and genetic effects (76,77). However, in recent years the role of oxidative stress induced by reactive oxygen species (ROS) generated by normal metabolic activity and lifestyle factors such as smoking, exercise and diet (Table 1) and the oxidative damage of important cellular biomolecules has been recognized as an important mechanism for the causation and progression of chronic diseases (Fig1) (11,13,22-23,34-35,48,51,54,67-68,92,95).

INTERNAL	EXTERNAL
Electron Transport System	Radiation
Lipid Oxidation	Air Pollutants
Respiratory Burst	Lifestyle Factors
Cytochromes P450	Diet

Table1: Reactive Oxygen Species (ROS) Formation

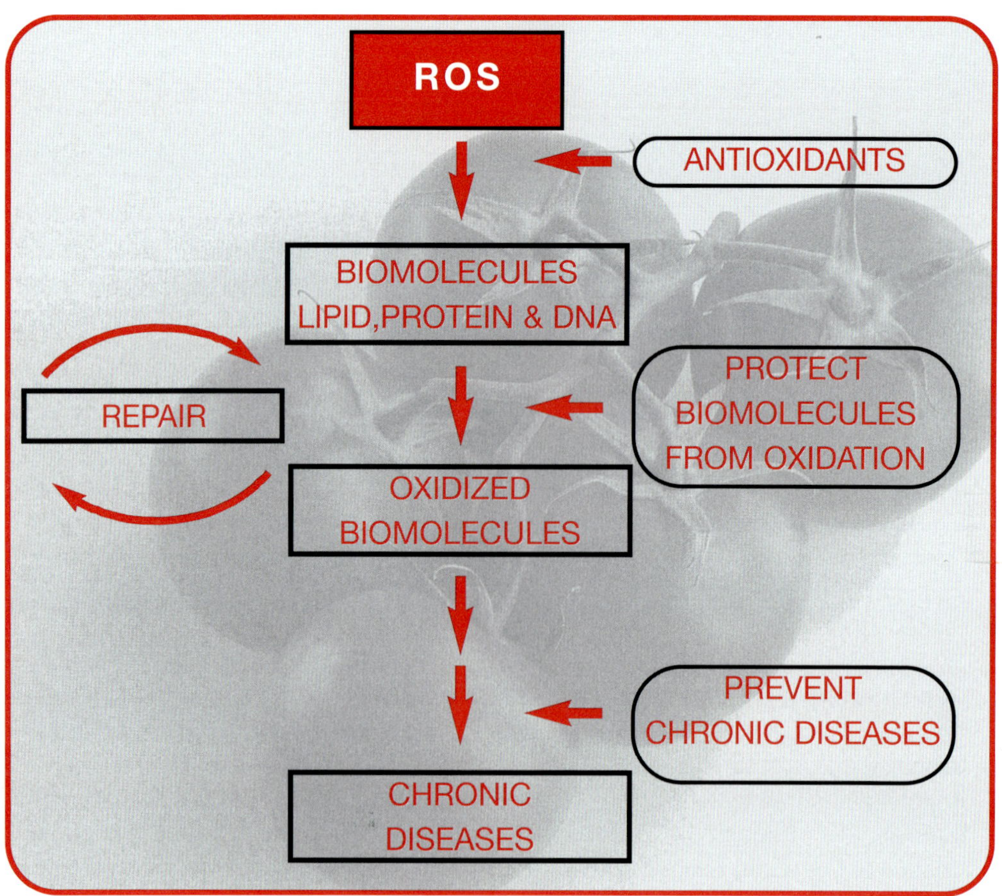

Fig1: Oxidative Stress and Chronic Diseases

Fruits and vegetables are a rich source of several beneficial compounds including antioxidants that can mitigate the damaging effect of ROS and provide cellular protection (Table 2).

Vitamins	Minerals	Phytochemicals
Folate	Magnesium	Carotenoids
Vitamin A	Potassium	Fiber (soluble & insoluble)
Vitamin C	Selenium	Flavonoids
Vitamin E		Indoles
Vitamin K		Isoflavoes
		Isothiocyanates
		Lignan
		Phytate
		Terpenoids (Saponins)

Table 2: Fruits and Vegetables: Some Potentially Beneficial Compounds

In addition to the traditional antioxidant vitamins such as vitamins A, E and C and minerals such as selenium, fruits and vegetables also contain several important phytonutrient antioxidants. The two important classes of phytonutrient antioxidants include fat soluble carotenoids and water soluble polyphenols. *In vitro* cell culture studies, laboratory animal studies, case control and cohort studies, and dietary intervention studies have all provided evidence in support of the role of antioxidants in the prevention of cancer and other chronic diseases. ß-carotene has long been recognized as an important carotenoid antioxidant having provitamin A activity (63). However, recent studies raised concerns regarding the safety of ß-carotene.

Another carotenoid antioxidant found naturally in plant foods is lycopene. Lycopene has received a great deal of attention as an effective antioxidant that can play an important role in reducing the risk of several chronic diseases (2-4,8,12,19-20,25,27,29-33,43-47,49-50,52,58-59,70,72,79,87).

Lycopene is a straight chain hydrocarbon containing 11 conjugated and 2 unconjugated double bonds and is an effective singlet oxygen quencher that is two times greater than ß-carotene and ten times greater than vitamin E (21,42). Lycopene is present in its natural, all transisomeric form in tomatoes. However, processing tomato into tomato products induces transformation to several cis isomers of lycopene, increasing its bioavailability (18,28,86).

The stability and antioxidant properties of lycopene have been studied in recent years. The 5-cis lycopene was shown to be the most stable form, having the highest antioxidant property (Fig 2) (16,61). Lycopene has been shown to be metabolized in the body by enzymatic and oxidative mechanisms (24,41,65,74).

I. CONFIGURATION STABILITY OF LYCOPENE ISOMERS ESTABLISHED AT TWO LEVELS OF AB INITIO COMPUTATIONS

5–*cis* > all-trans > 9–*cis* > 13–cis > 15–*cis* > 7–*cis* > 11–*cis*

II. ANTIOXIDANT PROPERTIES OF LYCOPENE ISOMERS AS INDICATED BY THEIR IONIZATION POTENTIALS

5–*cis* > 9–*cis* > 7–*cis* 13–cis > 15–*cis* > 11–*cis* > all-trans

Fig 2: Stability and Antioxidant Properties of Lycopene Isomers (16)

Unlike ß-carotene, lycopene lacks terminal cyclic rings and provitamin A properties. Animals and humans do not synthesize this important carotenoid and have to depend on dietary sources for their daily intake. Although lycopene is found naturally in fruits such as watermelon, pink guavas and pink grapefruits, tomatoes and processed tomato products constitute the major source of lycopene in human diet accounting for close to 90% of the total intake (79). The lycopene content of tomatoes and commonly consumed commercial tomato products is shown in Table 3.

Lycopene is the predominant carotenoid found in tomatoes followed by ß-carotene and other carotenoids (Fig 3) (1,71,89). It is also the major carotenoid present in human blood (14,69). Animal and human studies have shown that certain organs, such as the prostate, liver, brain and testicles preferentially accumulate lycopene, suggesting a specialized transportation mechanism for lycopene in these tissues (39). Epidemiological, cell culture, animal and human intervention studies have shown lycopene to be beneficial in the prevention of several human diseases. (Table 4) (9,26,30-33,39,60,62,64,73,78,80-84,90).

Group	Product	Lycopene (ppm) mean ±SEM, n=5
I. Fresh Tomatoes	Tomatoes	310.0 ± 4.6
II. Products for Food Preparation	Tomato Paste Tomato Puree Crushed Tomatoes	365.0 ± 3.6 195.6 ± 2.8 223.8 ± 0.9
III . Sauces	Tomato Sauce Spaghetti Sauce Pizza Sauce Seafood Sauce Chili Sauce	130.6 ± 1.2 191.2 ± 1.3 121.7 ± 0.8 185.6 ± 2.5 168.3 ± 1.6
IV. Condiments	Tomato Ketchup Light Ketchup Barbecue Sauce	123.9 ± 2.1 141.0 ± 2.1 42.9 ± 0.6
V. Readily Consumed	Tomato Juice Condensed Soup Ready to serve Soup Clam Cocktail Bloody Mary Mix	101.6 ± 0.6 72.7 ± 0.2 44.1 ± 0.6 43.3 ± 0.2 42.3 ± 0.3

Table 3: Lycopene Contents of Tomatoes and Commonly Consumed Commercial Tomato Products

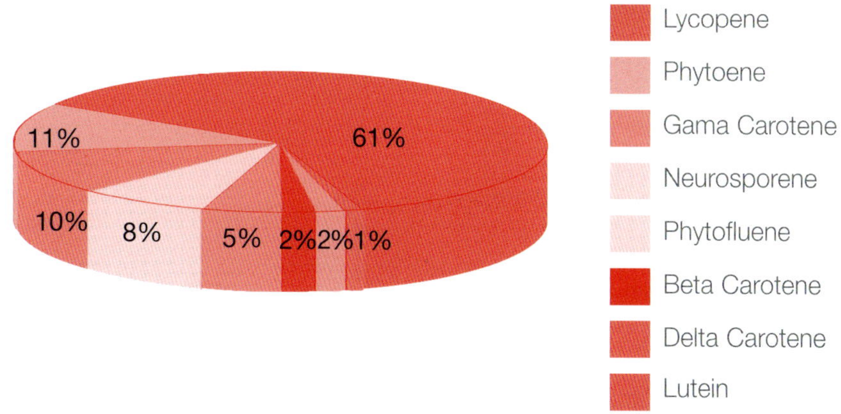

Fig 3: Carotenoid Profile of Tomato Products

Research shows that lycopene may reduce the risk of:

BREAST CANCER	CARDIOVASCULAR DISEASE
CERVICAL CANCER	AGING MACULAR DEGENERATION
PROSTATE CANCER	MALE INFERTILITY
SKIN CANCER	RADIATION DAMAGE
LUNG CANCER	ASTHMA.
COLON CANCER	OSTEOPOROSIS

Table 4: Health Benefits of Lycopene

Although most of the evidence in support of the beneficial role of lycopene in reducing the risk of chronic diseases is based on epidemiological studies, more recently, several clinical and dietary intervention studies are beginning to be undertaken. It is to be expected that results from these and other studies that are yet to be undertaken will enhance our knowledge about lycopene and disease prevention and perhaps even the treatment of some chronic diseases. They will also contribute to a better understanding of the mechanisms by which lycopene exerts its effect. Although the antioxidant mechanisms of lycopene in the prevention of human diseases has been the major focus of several studies, other mechanisms are also beginning to be recognized (Fig 4) (36-37,40,53,66,91,93-94).

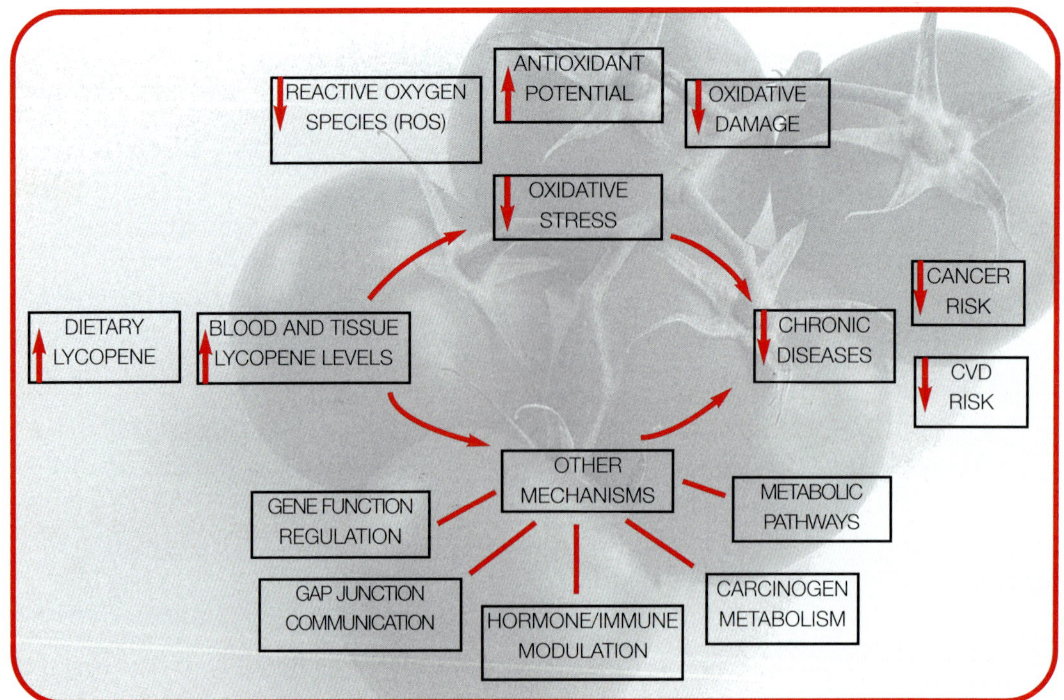

Fig 4: Proposed Mechanisms of Action of Lycopene

Evidence to date supports the beneficial role of lycopene in human health. Ongoing human intervention studies and other studies planned for the future will undoubtedly strengthen the existing scientific evidence. It will then be up to government agencies to allow appropriate health claims for lycopene and the food and related industries to use innovative strategies to promote the intake of lycopene that is consistent with maintaining good health.

REFERENCES:

1. Agarwal, A., Shen, H., Agarwal, S. and Rao, A. (2001) Lycopene content of tomato products: Its stability, bioavailability and in vivo antioxidant properties. *Journal of Medicinal Food* 4, 9-15.
2. Agarwal S and Rao AV (1988) Tomato lycopene and low density lipoprotein oxidation: A human dietary intervention study. *Lipids* 33, 981-984.
3. Agarwal S and Rao AV (2000) Tomato lycopene and its role in human health and chronic diseases. In *Canadian Medical Association Journal*, Vol. 163, pp. 739-44.
4. Agarwal S and Rao AV (2000.) Carotenoids and chronic diseases. *Drug Metabolism & Drug Interactions* 17, 189-210.
5. Ames BN, Gold LS and Willet WC (1996) Causes and prevention of cancer. *Proc Natl Acad Sci (USA)* 92, 5258-5265.
6. Ames BN, Shigenaga MK and TM., H. (1993) Oxidants, antioxidants and the degenerative diseases of aging. *Proc Natl Acad Sci USA* 90, 7915-7922.
7. Ansari MS and NP, G. (2003) A comparison of lycopene and orchidectomy vs orchidectomy alone in the management of advanced prostate cancer. *BJU International* 92, 375-378.
8. Arab L and Steck S (2000) Lycopene and cardiovascular disease. *Am J Clin Nutr* 71(suppl), 1691S-1695S.
9. Astrog P, Gradelet S, Berges R and Suschetet M (1997) Dietary lycopene decreases initiation of liver preneoplastic foci by diethylnitrosamine in rats. *Nutr Cancer* 29.

10. Aust, O., Ale-Agha, N., Zhang, L., Wollersen, H., Sies, H. and Stahl, W. (2003) Lycopene oxidation product enhances gap junction communication. *Food and Chemical toxicology* 41, 1399-1407.
11. Basu S, Michaelsson K, Olofsson H, Johansson S and Melhus H (2001) Association between oxidative stress and bone mineral density. *Biochemical & Biophysical Research Communications* 288, 275-279.
12. Bowen P, Chen L, Stacewicz-Sapuntzakis M, Duncan C, Sharifi R, Ghosh L, Kim HS, Christov-Tzelkov K and van Breemen R (2002) Tomato sauce supplementation and prostate cancer: lycopene accumulation and modulation of biomarkers of carcinogenesis. *Exp Biol Med (Maywood)* 227, 886-893.
13. Boyd NF and McGuire V (1990) Evidence of lipid peroxidation in premenopausal women with mammographic dysplasia. *Cancer Lett* 50, 31--37.
14. Brady WE, Mares-Perlman JA, Bowen P and Stacewicz- Sapuntzakis M (1997) Human serum carotenoid concentrations are related to physiologic and lifestyle factors. *J Nutr* 126, 129-137.
15. Britton G (1995) Structure and properties of carotenoids in relation to function. *FASEB J* 9, 1551-1558.
16. Chasse GA, Mak ML, Deretey E, Farkas I, Torday LL, Papp JG, DSarma DSR, Agarwal A, Chakravarthi S, Agarwal S and Rao AV (2001) An ab initio computational study on selected lycopene isomers. *J Mol Struc (Theochem)* 571, 27-37.
17. Chew, B. and Park, J. (2004) Carotenoid action on immune response. *Journal of Nutrition* 134, 257S-261S.
18. Clinton, S., Emenhoser, C. and Schwartz, S. (1996) Cis-trans lycopene isomers, carotenoids and retinol in human prostate. *Cancer Epidemiol Biomarkers Prev* 5, 823-833.
19. Clinton SK (1998) Lycopene: chemistry, biology, and implications for human health and disease. *Nutrition Reviews* 1, 35-51.
20. Cohen LA, Zhao Z, Pittman B and F, K. (1999) Effect of dietary lycopene on N-methylnitrosourea-induced mammary tumorigenesis. *Nutrition and Cancer* 34, 153-159.
21. Di Mascio P, Kaiser S and Sies H (1989) Lycopene as the most efficient biological carotenoid singlet oxygen quencher. *Arch Biochem Biophys* 274, 532-538.
22. Diaz M, Frei B, Vita JA and JF., K. (1997) Antioxidants and atherosclerotic heart disease. *N Engl J Med* 337, 408-416.
23. Ferrante RJ, Browne SE, Shinobu LA, Bowling AC, Baik MJ, MacGarvey U, Kowall NW, Brown RH Jr. and MF, B. (1997) Evidence of increased oxidative damage in both sporadic and familial amyotrophic lateral sclerosis. *J. Neurochem.* 69, 2064-2074.
24. Ferreira, D. (2004) Enzymatic and oxidative metabolites of lycopene. *Journal of Nutritional Biochemistry* 15, 493-502.
25. Franceschi S, Bidoli E, La Vecchia C, Talamini R, D'Avanzo B and E., N. (1994) Tomatoes and risk of digestive-tract cancers. *Int J Cancer* 59, 181-184.
26. Fuhramn B, Elis A and Aviram M (1997) Hypocholesterolemic effect of lycopene and ß-carotene is related to suppression of cholesterol synthesis and augmentation of LDL receptor activity in macrophage. *Biochem Biophys Res Commun* 233, 658-662.
27. Gann P, Ma J, Giovannucci E, Willett W, Sacks FM and Hennekens CH (1999) Lower prostate cancer risk in men with elevated plasma lycopene levels: results of a prospective analysis. *Cancer Res* 59, 1225-1230.
28. Gärtner C, Stahl W and Sies H (1997) Lycopene is more bioavailable from tomato paste than from fresh tomatoes. *Am J Clin Nutr*, 116-122.

29. Gerster H (1997) The potential role of lycopene for human health. *J Am Coll Nutr* 16, 109-126.
30. Giovannucci E (1999) Tomatoes, tomato-based products, lycopene, and cancer: review of the epidemiologic literature. *J National Cancer Institute* 91, 317-331.
31. Giovannucci E, Ascherio A, Rimm EB, Stampfer MJ, Colditz GA and Willett WC (1995) Intake of carotenoids and retinol in relation to risk of prostate cancer. *J Natl Cancer Inst* 87, 1767--76.
32. Giovannucci E, R. E., Liu Y, Stampfer MJ, Willett WC (2002) A prospective study of tomato products, lycopene, and prostate cancer risk. *Journal of the National Cancer Institute* 94, 391-398.
33. Gomez-Aracena J, Sloots J and Garcia-Rodriguez A et al (1997) Antioxidants in adipose tissue and myocardial infarction in Mediterranean area. The EURAMIC study in Malaga. *Nutr Metab Cardiovasc Dis* 7, 376-382.
34. Halliwell B, Cross CE and Gutteridge JMC (1992) Free radicals, antioxidants and human diseases: where are we now? *Journal of Laboratory and Clinical Medicine* 119, 598-620.
35. Halliwell B, Murcia MA, Chirico S and Aruoma OI (1995) Free radicals and antioxidants in food and in vivo: what they do and how they work. *Crit Rev Food Sci Nutr* 35, 7-20.
36. Heber, D. (2002) Mechanisms of action of lycopene: Overview. In *Lycopene and the prevention of chronic diseases*, Vol. 1, Rao, A. and D, H. eds, pp. 41-42. Caledonian Science Press, Scotland.
37. Heber D and Lu Q-L (2002) Overview of Mechanisms of Action of Lycopene. *Exp Biol Med (Maywood)* 227, 920-923.
38. Heller FR, Descamps O and Hondekijn JC (1998) LDL oxidation: therapeutic perspectives. *Atherosclerosis* 137, S25-S31.
39. Jain CK, Agarwal S and Rao AV (1999) The effect of dietary lycopene on bioavailability, tissue distribution, in-vivo antioxidant properties and colonic preneoplasia in rats. *Nutr Res* 19, 1383-1391.
40. Karas M, Amir H, Fishman D, Danilenko M, Segal S, Nahum A, Koifmann A, Giat Y, Levy J and Sharoni Y (2000) Lycopene Interferes with Cell Cycle Progression and Insulin-Like Growth Factor I Signaling in Mammary Cancer Cells. *Nutrition and Cancer* 36, 101-111.
41. Khachik F, Beecher GR and Smith JC Jr (1995) Lutein, lycopene and their oxidative metabolite in chemo prevention of cancer. *J Cell Biochem* Suppl 22, 236-246.
42. Khachik F, Carvallo L, Bernstein PS, Muir GJ, Zhao DY and Katz NB (2002) Chemistry, distribution and metabolism of tomato carotenoids and their impact on human health. *Exp Biol Med (Maywood)* 227, 845-851.
43. Kim DJ, Takasuka N, Nishino H and H, T. (2000) Chemo prevention of lung cancer by lycopene. *Biofactors* 13, 95-102.
44. Kim L, Rao AV and LG., R. (2002) Effect of lycopene on Prostate LNCaP Cancer Cells in Culture. *Journal of Medicinal Food* 5, 181-187.
45. Kim L, Rao AV and Rao LG (2003) Lycopene II - Effect on osteoblasts: The caroteroid lycopene stimulates cell proliferation and alkaline phosphatase activity of SaOS-2 cells. *J Med Food* 6, 79-86.
46. Kohlmeier L and Hastings SB (1995) Epidemiologic evidence of a role of carotenoids in cardiovascular disease prevention. *Am J Clin Nutr* 62(Suppl), 1370S-1376S.
47. Kohlmeier L, Kark JD, Gomez-Garcia E, Martin BC, Steck SE, Kardinaal AFM, Ringstad J, Thamm M, Masaev V, Riemersma R, Martin-Moreno JM, Huttunen JK and Kok F (1997) Lycopene and myocardial infarction risk in the EURAMIC study. *Am J Epidemiol* 146, 618-626.

48. Kristenson M and al., e. (1997) Antioxidant state and mortality from coronary heart disease in Lithuanian and Swedish men: concomitant cross sectional study of men aged 50. *BMJ* 314, 629--33.
49. Kucuk O, Sarkar FH and Sakr W, e. a. (2001) Phase II randomized clinic trial of lycopene supplementation before radical prostatectomy. *Cancer Epidemiol Biomarkers Prev* 10, 861-8.
50. Kucuk, O., Sarkar, F., Djuric, Z., Sakr, W., Pollak, M., Khachik, F.,] Banerjee, M., Bertram, J. and Wood DP, J. (2002) Effects of lycopene supplementation in patients with localized prostate cancer. *Experimental Biology and Medicine* 227, 881-885.
51. Lassegue B and KK, G. (2004) Reactive oxygen species in hypertension. *American Journal of Hypertension* 17, 852-860.
52. LaVecchia C (1997) Mediterranean epidemiological evidence on tomatoes and the prevention of digestive tract cancers. *Proc Soc Exp Bio Med* 218, 125--128.
53. Livny O, Kaplan I, Reifen R, Polak-Charcon S, Madar Z and B, S. (2002) Lycopene inhibits proliferation and enhances gap-junction communication of KB-1 human oral tumor cells. *Journal of Nutrition* 132, 3754-3759.
54. Loft S and Poulsen HE (1996.) Cancer risk and oxidative DNA damage in man. *J Mol Med* 74, 297-312.
55. Matulka, R., Hood, A. and Griffiths, J. (2004) Safety evaluation of a natural tomato oleoresin extract derived from food-processing tomatoes. *Regulatory Toxicology and Pharmacology* 39, 390-402.
56. McClain, R. and Bausch, J. (2003) Summary of safety studies conducted with synthetic lycopene. *Regul Pharmacol Toxicol* 37, 274-285.
57. Mills PK, Beeson WL, Phillips RL and GE, F. (1989) Cohort study of diet, lifestyle, and prostate cancer in Adventist men. *Cancer Epidemiol Biomarkers Prev* 64, 598-604.
58. Mohanty NK, Kumar R and Gupta NP (2001) Lycopene therapy in the management of idiopathic oligoasthenospermia. *Ind J Urol* 56, 102-103..
59. Morris DL, Kritchevsky and Davis CE (1994) Serum carotenoids and coronary heart disease: the Lipid Research Clinics Coronary Primary Prevention Trial and Follow-up Study. *JAMA* 272, 1439-1441.
60. Narisawa T, Fukaura Y, Hasebe M, Nomura S, Oshima S, Sakamoto H, Inakuma T, Ishiguro Y, Takayasu J and H, N. (1998) Prevention of N-methylnitrosourea-induced colon carcinogenesis in F344 rats by lycopene and tomato juice rich in lycopene. *Japanese Journal of Cancer Research* 89, 1003-1008.
61. Nguyen, M. and Schwartz, S. (1998) Lycopene stability during food processing. *Proceedings of the Society for Experimental Biology and Medicine* 218, 101-105.
62. Okajima E, Tsutsumi M, Ozono S, Akai H, Denda A, Nishino H, Oshima S, Sakamoto H and Y, K. (1998) Inhibitory effect of tomato juice on rat urinary bladder carcinogenesis after N-butyl-N-(4hydroybutyl) nitrosamine initiation. *Japanese Journal of Cancer Research* 89, 22-26.
63. Paiva, S. and Ressell, R. (1999) Beta carotene and other carotenoids as antioxidants. *J Am Coll Nutrition* 18, 426-433.
64. Paran E and Engelhard Y (2001) Effect of Lyc-O-Mato, standardized tomato extract on blood pressure, serum lipoproteins, plasma homocysteine and oxidative stress markers in grade 1 hypertensive patients. *Proceedings of the 16th Annual Scientific Meeting of the Society of Hypertension, San Francisco, USA).*
65. Parker RS (1996) Absorption, metabolism and transport of carotenoids. *FASEB J* 10, 542-551.

66. Parthasarathy S (1998) Mechanisms by which dietary antioxidants may prevent cardiovascular diseases. *J Med Food* 1, 45-51.
67. Parthasarathy S, Steinberg D and Witztum JL (1992) The role of oxidized low-density lipoproteins in pathogenesis of atherosclerosis. *Ann Rev Med* 43, 219-225.
68. Pincemail J (1995) *Free radicals and antioxidants in human disease*. Birkh user Verlag, Basel.
69. Polidori MC, Stahl W, Eichler O, Niestroj I and Sies H (2001) Profiles of antioxidants in human plasma. *Free Rad Biol Med* 30, 456-462.
70. Rao, A. and Rao, L. (2004) Lycopene and human health. *Current Topics in Nutraceutical Research* 2, 127-136.
71. Rao, A., Waseem, Z. and Agarwal, S. (1999) Lycopene content of tomatoes and tomato products and their contribution to dietary lycopene. *Food Research International* 31, 737-741.
72. Rao AV (2002a) Lycopene, tomatoes and health: New perspectives 2000. In *Lycopene and the prevention of chronic diseases: Major findings from five international conferences*, AV, R. and D, H. eds, pp. 19-28. Caledonian Science Press, Scotland.
73. Rao AV (2002b) Lycopene, tomatoes and the prevention of coronary heart disease. *Exp Bio Med* 227, 908-913.
74. Rao AV and Agarwal S (1998a) Bioavailability and in vivo antioxidant properties of lycopene from tomato products and their possible role in the prevention of cancer. *Nutr Canc* 31, 199-203.
75. Rao AV and Agarwal S (1998b) Effect of diet and smoking on serum lycopene and lipid peroxidation. *Nutr Res* 18, 713-721.
76. Rao AV and Agarwal S (1999) Role of lycopene as antioxidant carotenoid in the prevention of chronic diseases: a review. *Nutrition Research* 19, 305-323.
77. Rao AV and Agarwal S (2000) Role of antioxidant lycopene in cancer and heart disease. *Journal of the American College of Nutrition* 19, 563-569.
78. Rao AV and Balachandran B (2003) Role of oxidative stress and antioxidants in neurodegenerative diseases. *Nutritional Neurosciences* 5, 291-309.
79. Rao AV, Fleshner N and Agarwal S (1999) Serum and tissue lycopene and biomarkers of oxidation in prostate cancer patients: a case-control study. *Nutrition and Cancer* 33, 159-162.
80. Rao AV and Shen HL (2002) Effect of low dose lycopene intake on lycopene bioavailability and oxidative stress. *Nutr Res*, 1125-1131.
81. Rao LG, Collins ES, Josse RG, Strauss A and Rao AV (2005) Lycopene consumption significantly decreases oxidative stress and bone resorption marker in postmenopausal women at risk of osteoporosis. *Joint Meeting of the ECTS and IBMS* June 25-29. Geneva, Switzerland.
82. Rao LG, Krishnadev N, Banasikowska K and Rao AV (2003) Lycopene I - Effect on osteoclasts: Lycopene inhibits basal and parathyroid hormone-stimulated osteoclast formation and mineral resorption mediated by reactive oxygen species in rat bone marrow cultures. *J Med Food* 6, 69-78.
83. Rocchi E, Borghi A, Paolillo F, Pradelli M and G, C. (1991) Carotenoids and liposoluble vitamins in liver cirrhosis. *Journal of Laboratory and Clinical Medicine* 118, 176-185.
84. Sharoni Y, Giron E, Rise M and J, L. (1997) Effects of lycopene-enriched tomato oleoresin on 7,12-dimethyl-benz[a]anthracene-induced rat mammary tumors. *Cancer Detect Prev* 21, 118-123.

85. Stadtman ER (1992) Protein oxidation and aging. ***Science*** 257, 1220-1224.
86. Stahl W and Sies H (1992) Uptake of lycopene and its geometrical isomers is greater from heat-processed than from unprocessed tomato juice in humans. ***J Nutr*** 122, 2161-2166.
87. Stahl W and Sies H (1996) Lycopene: a biologically important carotenoid for humans? ***Arch Biochem Biophys*** 336, 1-9.
88. Street DA, Comstock GW and Salkeld RM et al (1994) Serum antioxidant and myocardial infarction: are low levels of carotenoids and alpha-tocopherol risk factors for myocardial infarction? ***Circulation*** 90, 1154-1161.
89. U.S. Department of Agriculture and Agricultural Research Service. 1998. USDA-NCC Carotenoid database for U.S. Foods. 1998 (1998) Nutrient Data Laboratory Home Page
90. Venkateswaran, V., Fleshner, N., Sugar, L. and Klotz, L. (2004) Antioxidants block prostate cancer in lady transgenic mice. ***Cancer Research*** 64, 5891-5896.
91. Wertz, K., Siler, U. and Goralczyk, R. (2004) Lycopene: modes of action to promote prostate health. ***Archives of Biochemistry and Biophysics*** 430, 127-134.
92. Witztum JL (1994) The oxidation hypothesis of artherosclerosis. ***Lancet .*** 344, 793-796.
93. Zhang LX, Cooney RV and Bertram JS (1991) Carotenoids enhance gap junctional communication and inhibit lipid peroxidation in C3H/10T1/2 cells: relationship to their cancer chemo preventive action. ***Carcinogenesis*** 12, 2109-2114.
94. Zhang L-X, Cooney RV and Bertram JS (1992) Carotenoids up-regulate connexin43 gene expression independent of their provitamin A or antioxidant properties. ***Cancer Res*** 52, 5707-5712.
95. Zock P and Katan MB (1998) Diet, LDL oxidation, and coronary artery disease. ***Am J Clin Nutr*** 68, 759-760.

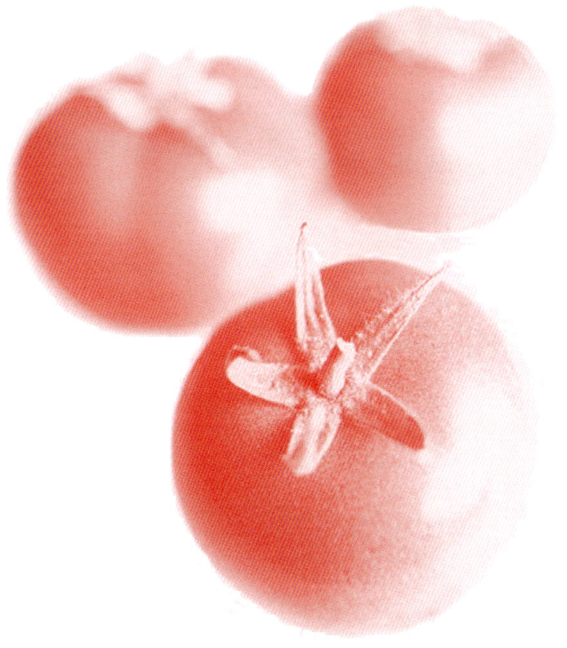

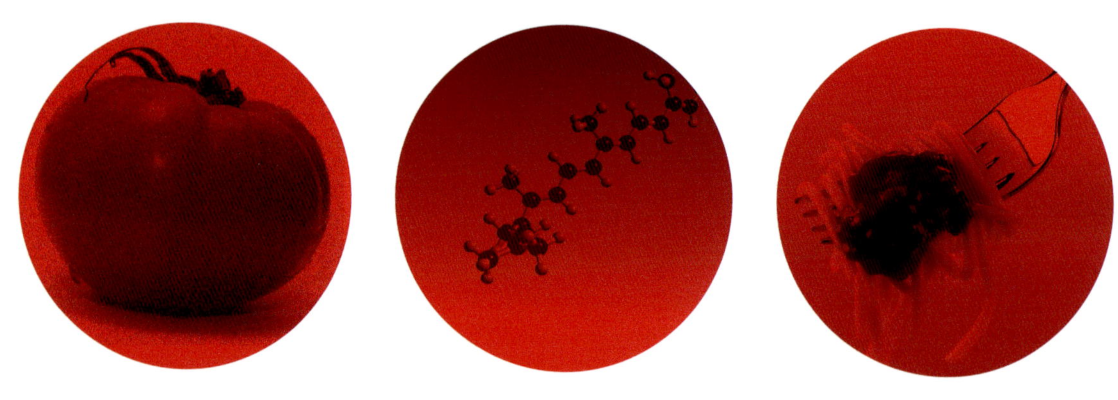

Content, Behaviour and Bioavailability of Lycopene in Processed Tomatoes

Dr. Carlo Leoni
SSICA – Experimental Station for The Food Preserving Industry
Parma, Italy

Abstract

At present, consumer's attitudes towards health include renewed attention to the hygienic and dietary aspects of foods, i.e. their *nutritional qualities*, and also the supposed antioxidant activities of some food components.

A basic idea on which all nutritional scientists agree is that increased consumption of diets rich and varied in fruit and vegetables will improve the health of almost any human population, providing protection from certain pathologies correlated to oxidative processes. This diet (of which the Mediterranean diet is the best example), is known to be beneficial for health especially with regard to the development of chronic degenerative diseases (1, 2). Vegetable products contain many substances which may have beneficial effects on health. Tomato is one of the most used vegetables in the Mediterranean diet. Epidemiological studies have demonstrated that tomato consumption provides a protective effect against some types of cancers and ischaemic heart disease. This protective effect has mainly been ascribed to the antioxidant activity of some tomato components. Therefore, tomatoes appear especially important in terms of public health since they are consumed in large quantities and are rich in several compounds believed to protect or reduce the risk for chronic degenerative diseases (3).

The antioxidant composition of tomatoes is complex and rich, and optimisation criteria of processing and storage technologies should take into account the preservation of the whole antioxidant pool and of its functional properties. Tomato is a source of several microcomponents with antioxidant properties (carotenoids, vitamins, folates, polyphenolic compounds, tocopherols) like many other fruits and vegetables even if in much lower concentrations (4). Carotenoids are among the first compounds to have attracted the attention of scientists to the effects of fruits and vegetables, and tomatoes are especially rich in one of them: the typically red-coloured carotenoid, lycopene. Tomatoes are the main dietary source of lycopene, present in tomatoes and in few other fruits and vegetables.

Lycopene in tomato products has always been considered very important, although until the '80s the interest in it was confined to its characteristic as a red pigment and thus responsible for the red colour of tomato products. A bright red colour, typical of the mature raw tomato, is taken as evidence of quality by processors and consumers alike and colour has been recognised by regulatory authorities in establishing standards of quality. In the last two decades, this red pigment has also been seen as a possible natural antioxidant compound, with promising implications for human nutrition and health.

It is important to note that a large proportion of tomatoes are eaten in the form of industrially-processed products. Tomatoes can be easily processed into several products which are consumed in large amounts, and during this processing, the main components of tomatoes are preserved and even concentrated. Because of this widespread and large consumption, tomatoes appear as one of the most interesting foods in terms of global health.

The tomato is now the most important vegetable product used in the making of industrial preserves. The "traditional" tomato-growing nations are the USA, Italy, Greece, Spain, Portugal, Turkey, the countries of North Africa, Israel, Canada, Mexico, Chile and Brazil and, more recently, China, the southern republics of the former USSR, Australia and India. Although tomato processing is an industry which produces products of relatively low added value, the USA (in particular California) and the Mediterranean countries alone process 70% of the world's entire tomato production.

Between 25 and 30 million tons of tomatoes are processed each year, more than a third of the 70 millions tons produced each year. The average per capita consumption of processed tomato products is nearly 3.5 kg (on a fresh tomato basis), with variations from zero for at least three quarters of world population to 14-15 kg in the EU, and to more than 30 kg in Italy and the USA.

Processed tomatoes and in particular tomato paste have always been considered "poor" products with a low added value destined for being used as a basis for more elaborated products (sauces, ketchup), both for domestic and industrial trade purposes: semi-processed products dominated by the "price" rather than finished products with their own dignity linked, in particular, to intrinsic quality factors.

These findings introduce novel optimisation criteria and goals for processed tomato products. These products are an important food from the sensory point of view offering a good service quality, and with positive effects on the prevention of the most important and common diseases of our modern world should receive, if only because of their affordability, greater attention from consumers and the media.

If it is clear that the starting point for the optimisation of tomato nutritional properties is raw material, great attention must also be paid to avoid or minimise the detrimental effects induced by technological processing and by the storage of processed products.

Data and information supplied by scientific literature on lycopene degradation during common tomato processing such as heat sterilisation, concentration by evaporation and dehydration and also for storage of processed tomato products, though sometimes inconsistent or not completely clear, allow for some general conclusions and comments. Since the operating conditions applied to the tests are either not well defined or do not correspond to those used for industrial treatments, the results should be considered as being often unreliable.

The data seem to suggest that lycopene is stable to heat treatments for tomato concentration and cooking and also during processed tomato storage. The stability is lower for products submitted to treatments which have damaged the cell walls and which have consequently reduced the protective effect concerning lycopene *coagula* (lycopene in hydrophobic products and in aqueous matrix is in this microform). Researchers substantially agree in considering this compound stable to processing, in terms of both degradation and isomerisation rate. Even air-drying, which is a very severe treatment in terms of oxidative stress, does not cause serious lycopene losses (5,6,7). Some of the studies reviewed witnessed a relatively high lycopene loss and isomerisation in heat-treated tomato products; a possible reason for these results, which are in contrast with other data, could be the differing analytical methods and procedures that were applied. On the contrary, lycopene is much less stable towards isomerisation and oxidation when it is solubilised in organic solvent (or in the presence of lipids).

Fair Concerted Action 97-3233 made an assessment of the available literature which seems to indicate that lycopene is relatively stable during heat-treatments, that it possesses a fair stability during storage, with only slight reductions under severe oxidative conditions such as hot-air drying and a light discoloration during deep freezing (6). But a lot of research does lead to contradictory conclusions as to the supposed marked degradation effect of storage, probably due to the fact that lycopene was frequently measured in second-stage tomato products, with high oil/fat percentages (sauces) and facilitated partial solubilisation of lycopene and subsequent higher reactivity and degradation.

It seemed interesting therefore to report the results of the effects of storage conditions on the lycopene content of tomato purees obtained by different processing techniques, summarising the trials conducted using a pilot plant by Tamburini et al. (8). Samples of tomato puree were prepared first by extracting the juice, according to the conventional technique, varying extraction temperature (extraction of juice with cold-break and hot break techniques) and pulper hole size. The samples obtained were subjected to different storage conditions and the changes in lycopene content were monitored over a 12-month period. In this way, six kinds of tomato puree with different physical characteristics (consistency, colour and granulometry) were obtained. All in all, no difference occurs with the different processing techniques applied, at least under the conditions tested.

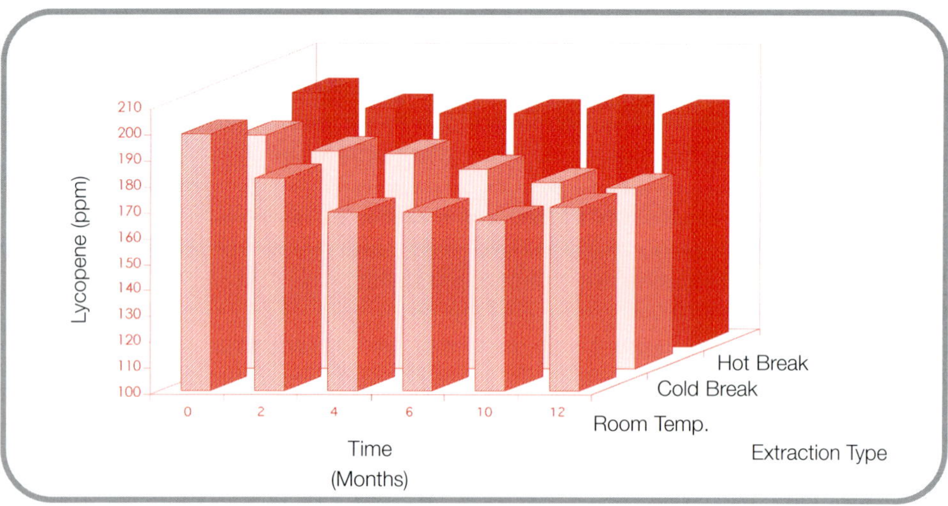

Fig 1: Lycopene content during storage of tomato passata obtained with different juice extraction methods.

A detailed analysis of the changes occurring over time in the samples prepared under different temperature conditions reveals that hot break, though typically involving blanching at high temperature (more than 90°C) for some dozens of seconds (which could make one suppose it would cause a considerable decrease in lycopene content) actually lessens lycopene levels only to a limited extent, but that it seems to preserve the pigment over time better than either cold break or extraction at room temperature (Fig.1). During storage, lycopene is better maintained in the hot break-treated product. As a result of the enzyme-inactivating hot break process (which keeps the tomato cells more intact, resulting in more difficult oxidative attacks) lycopene content in the hot break treated samples remains nearly unchanged even after 12 months of storage, whereas little variations in lycopene content occur in the cold break treated samples.

The other effects analysed (diameter of the pulper holes and storage temperature) cause no significant, technologically interesting variations in lycopene content. The results of the experience reported lead us to state that when lycopene remains within the original hydrophilic matrix and most of all, within a whole cell, it is considerably stable but, because of the subsequent scarce reactivity, it probably presents lower bioavailability and therefore it could be practically ineffective in realising its potential antioxidant activity.
The study of the effect of the industrial operations for the preparation of tomato powders on lycopene content and on colour carried out by Cabassi *et. al*.(7) substantially highlighted a moderate loss (5%) of total lycopene content which can be traced back to isomerisation and oxidation phenomena.

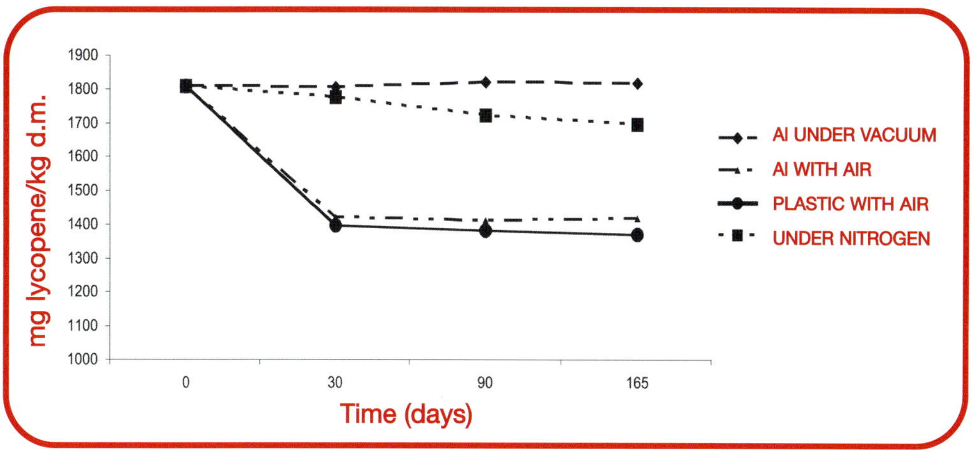

Fig 2: Decrease in total lycopene over time related to different types of package

The comparison of lycopene content in different flexible packaging materials showed that the highest preservation of lycopene was obtained with vacuum-packaging in Al/polythene pouches (Fig.2). A very good result was also given by N_2-packaging in polymer (PE and PVA) trays sealed with a PET film. In the packages containing air (and therefore oxygen) lycopene loss was decidedly higher (22-25%). Storage time showed a significant effect, which was reflected in an average 13% decrease in total lycopene in the samples during the first month of storage. However, it must be observed that this average value is the result of moderate decreases in vacuum and N_2-packaging (2%) and more pronounced ones in packaging in the presence of air (24%). The more marked effect found during the first month of storage of the powders suggests that a lycopene portion, probably that present on the air-exposed surface, is more sensitive to the action of oxidants compared with that inside the granules themselves.

With regard to freezing action, tomato products kept at temperatures suitable for frozen storage undergo a decrease in the concentration of the characteristic red pigment, lycopene, and a parallel loss in colour. The results show an interesting similarity with what has been described about tomato powders. Loss took place mainly during the first 50 days, and the properties were then substantially maintained for longer storage times. In products packaged in low oxygen barrier material and kept in cardboard outer packaging, loss continued. Average lycopene loss was around 18.5% after 50 days and 20.6% after 150 days (Fig.3).

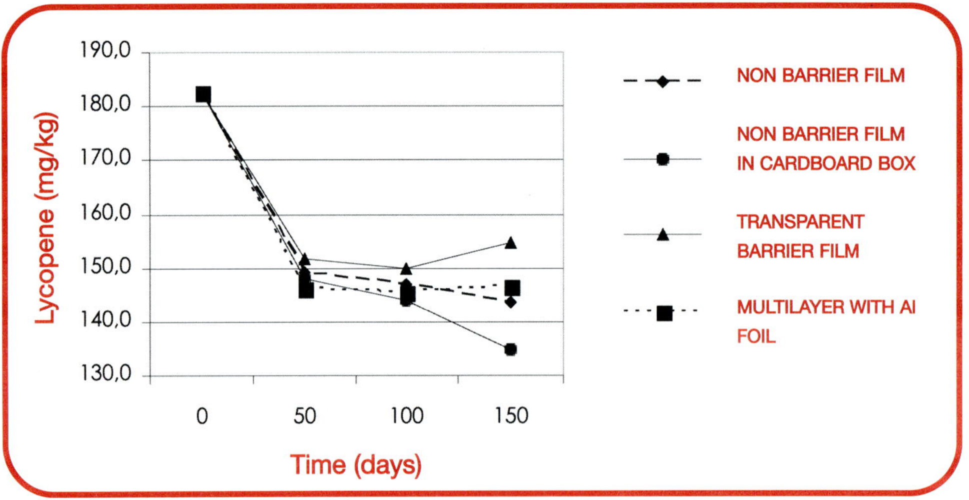

Fig 3: Lycopene decrease over time on the basis of the type of packaging

The presence of oil proved a detrimental condition for the maintenance of lycopene and of colour, leading to a lycopene loss of around 30%, compared to 13% in puree without oil. The combination "product with oil in a non-barrier packaging in cardboard box" proved the most detrimental to the maintenance of colour and lycopene content parameters (9).

In formulated products (i.e. frozen pizzas), lycopene behaviour confirms that found by Cremona, with higher differences probably caused by a higher ratio between exposed surface and weight of tomato products. There was a practically zero reduction in lycopene concentration in the oxygen-barrier packaging compensated with N_2, whereas in the non-O_2 barrier packaging there was a 29% decrease; a stronger negative effect was found when the product was inserted in cardboard secondary package (10).

Lycopene content must be distinguished from lycopene bioavailability. Also, the above mentioned studies are incomplete because they only aimed at measuring the lycopene content and not its bioavailability, which is most important for the nutritional quality of the product. The most stimulating objective of the research on lycopene is, perhaps, to evaluate the actual bioavailability for humans in the forms in which it is present in processed tomato products (11).

Although there are a number of comparative studies on the bioavailability of lycopene in tomato products, there are no proven methods for the quantitative assessment of carotenoid bioavailability, even of ß-carotene which has been the most frequently studied. A few studies have been carried out on the bioavailability of lycopene in the human diet. Some of them indicate that the absorption of lycopene is greater from heat-treated tomato juice than from untreated juice, and others indicate that absorption from tomato paste is higher than from fresh tomatoes.

It has been clearly demonstrated that the physical state and processing history of a food item has a very marked effect on the availability of these compounds for absorption. This indicates that disruption of the food matrix and thermal history via processing technique could be the most important factor affecting bioavailability. It is also known that the bioavailability of carotenoids is markedly affected by the fat content of the general diet, since the presence of lipids is essential for the extraction of carotenoids from the aqueous bulk of the food and for the formation of mixed micelles via which the carotenoids are then absorbed by enterocytes and transferred to the tissues (via plasma lipoproteins). Carotenoids are passively absorbed lipophilic compounds and their bioavailability is therefore affected by those factors that influence the mass transfer of the carotenoids from the food into the mixed micelles that can be absorbed by the intestine. Carotenoids are passively absorbed along with lipids. The efficiency of absorption of the carotenoids is, therefore, dependent on the release of lipophilic molecules and crystals of carotenoids from the food microstructure and their dissolution into dietary lipids during processing or domestic preparation, and during the digestive process. It is now recognised that release and dissolution are the most important factors governing carotenoid bioavailability; so it is not surprising to find greater lycopene bioavailability from heat-treated tomato products that have been homogenised or co-processed with oils: absorption can be improved by cooking and homogenising the food, thus breaking down the cell structure, as long as the cooking is carried out in the presence of oil or fat. The lycopene, as long as it remains in the aqueous matrix and, particularly, inside the undamaged cells is very stable and only slightly reactive: its bioavailability is therefore scarce and its efficacy as an antioxidant almost zero.

Conversely, when lycopene solubilises in a lipophilic matrix, it is considerably reactive and more available; therefore, it could suitably perform its antioxidant activity. Its assimilation is decidedly better if foods are cooked and homogenised so as to disrupt cells and even more if it occurs in the presence of oils or fats. However, it is obvious that this higher reactivity makes lycopene much more unprotected against the degradation activity of environmental conditions (air, biological matrix components, temperature).

In conclusion, it has been demonstrated that tomato processed products can be an important source of lycopene consumption. This is true in quantitative terms because the amounts of lycopene in tomatoes are higher than those in fresh fruit which, in addition, is frequently eaten before it is completely ripe, when the lycopene has not yet reached optimum levels. It is also true in qualitative terms, i.e. in a more available form. The preparation of sauces in the presence of oil or fat allows lycopene to be solubilised (particularly if the molecule has no physical defences, i.e. whole cell walls). Such processing makes it more readily available for humans.

It is also important to remember that, if lycopene in an aqueous matrix is very stable and therefore able to keep its potential for a long time, it is much more reactive in a lipid-rich matrix and thus more available, but also much more easily degradable. In journalistic terms: enjoy tomato sauces regularly, but prepare them using tomato products, not forgetting olive oil and, preferably, just before consumption.

REFERENCES:

1. Corpet DE, Gerber M, 'Alimentation méditérranéenne et Santé. I-caractéristiques. Maladies cardio-vasculaires et autres affections', Méd Nut, 1997 4, 129-42.
2. Gerber M, Corpet DE 'Alimentation méditérranéenne et Santé. II-Cancers'. Méd Nut, 1997 4, 143-54.
3. Leoni C, Bartholin G, Giovanelli G and van Boekel T in Grolier P,. Leoni C, Gerber M and Bilton R, The white book on antioxidants in tomatoes and tomato products and their health benefits, Chapter 2, 2-47 CMITI, Avignon, 2001, ISSN 1145-9565.
4. Leoni C 'Improving the nutritional quality of processed fruits and vegetables: the case of tomatoes" in Fruit and vegetable processing - Improving quality - ed. Wim Jongen - Woodhead Publishing Limited Abington, 2002 ISBN 1 85573 548 2
5. Lovric T, Sablek Z, Boskovic M, 'Cis-trans isomerisation of lycopene and colour stability of foam-mat dried tomato powder during storage' J. Sci. Food Agric., 1970 21, 641-47.
6. Zanoni B, Peri C, Nani R, Lavelli V. 'Oxidative heat damage of tomato halves as affected by drying' Food Res. Int., 1998 31, 395-401.
7. Cabassi A, Sandei L and Leoni C, 'Effects of industrial operations and storage conditions on colour and carotenoids of tomato powders', Ind Conserve, 2001, 76 299-313.
8. Tamburini R, Sandei L, Aldini A, De Sio F and Leoni C., 'Effect of storage conditions on lycopene content in tomato purees obtained with different processing techniques' Ind. Conserve, 1999, 74 341-57.
9. Cremona F, Sandei L, Taddei C, Leoni C-'Evaluation of the effects over time of freezing on lycopene content and on colour of frozen tomato products' Ind. Conserve, 2004, 79, 379-395
10. Taddei C, Sandei L, Cremona F, Leoni C- 'Evaluation of the effects over time of freezing on lycopene content and on colour of frozen pizzas surface' Ind. Conserve, 2005, 80, 235-256
11. Faulks R, Southon S, Böhm V and Porrini M. in Grolier P,. Leoni C, Gerber M and Bilton R, The white book on antioxidants in tomatoes and tomato products and their health benefits, Chapter 2, 48-73 CMITI, Avignon, 2001, ISSN 1145-9565.
12. Parker,R S, 'Bioavailability of carotenoids', Eur. J. Clin. Nutr., 1997, 51-Suppl 1. S86-S90.

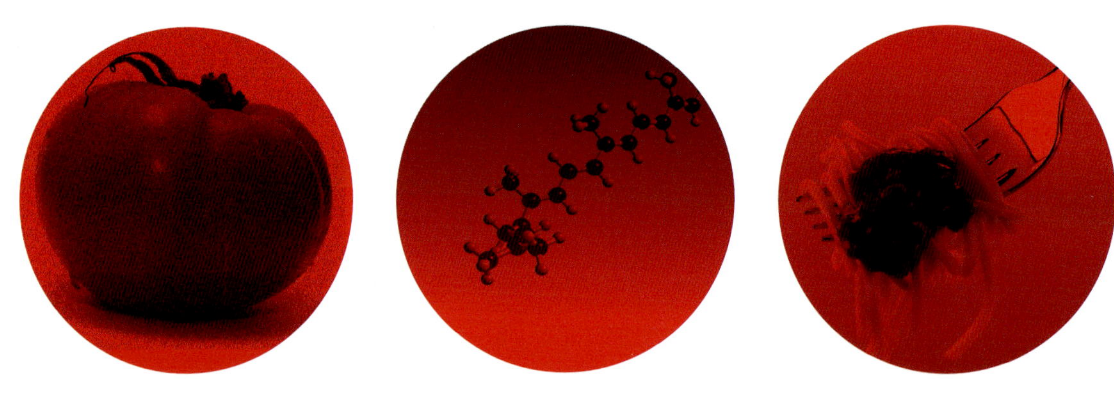

Lycopene Analysis in Foods

Dr. Montaña Cámara
Dr. M.C. Sánchez Mata
Department of Nutrition and Bromotology II
Faculty of Pharmacy,
Complutense University,
Madrid, Spain

Abstract

The knowledge of lycopene content in foods is the first step towards studying its role in diet and health. Recent advances in analytical methods have enabled updating and expansion of carotenoid databases. Lycopene differs from other carotenoids in its physicochemical properties. Due to its solubility and instability, it is necessary to carefully handle lycopene during its purification and analysis to avoid its degradation and isomerization. In this chapter, a review of the literature is reported. Methods for the efficient extractation of lycopene from food samples are reported, which take into account the importance of sample preparation, the selection of the extraction solvent, the extraction procedure (with special emphasis on saponification as a possible way to improve the extraction). The identification and quantification of lycopene can be done with different methods: HPLC, spectrophotometry, or colour evaluation, which are described in this chapter. Lycopene also plays a crucial role in biological systems as a potent oxygen radicals scavenger. The evaluation of fruit antioxidant capacity is not a simple task; most of the methods for the total antioxidant activity (TAA) are generally based on the inhibition of certain reactions by the presence of antioxidants. Many of these methods, based on the removal of generated free radicals by the presence of antioxidants, have also been reviewed.

INTRODUCTION

The knowledge of precise lycopene content in foods is the first step toward establishing its role in relation to diet and health. Although, because of some inherent difficulties, carotenoid analysis is not an easy task. However, tangible improvements in analytical methodology and instrumentation have been achieved in recent years(1).

Carotenoids are non-polar compounds, insoluble in water and soluble in organic solvents. Lycopene is soluble in chloroform, benzene, ethyl ether, petroleum ether or hexane, and it is almost insoluble in ethanol and methanol. This compound is highly instable to light, heat, atmospheric oxygen and metals such as Fe or Cu, which makes its preservation and analysis in complex samples such as foods difficult. It often undergoes degradation, formation of stereoisomers, structural rearrangements and other physicochemical reactions. The main mechanisms of lycopene losses are oxidation and isomerization of all-*trans*-form to *cis*-isomers (2-4).

Efficient analysis methods are particularly useful for the determination of this compound, due to its characteristics of solubility and instability, which makes a very carefully handling process and short time analysis necessary to avoid degradation and isomerization of lycopene. For this reason, the analytical methods for lycopene in vegetables are limited and the necessity for a reliable and rapid analysis method for lycopene in vegetable products is recognised (5, 6).

LYCOPENE EXTRACTION FROM FOOD SAMPLES

Extraction of analytes from a sample matrix is one of the most important parts of the analysis, since accuracy and specifity of the method is directly related to the efficacy of extraction and the presence of interferences in the extract that will be analyzed. Other components in the matrix may influence the extraction and quantification of carotenoids. Foods are variable and complex matrices, which usually require long and complex treatments, several extraction steps, and an efficient purification to avoid undesirable interferences during the analysis. Knowledge of the sample matrix is critical for accurate quantification, as many factors regarding the food matrix must be considered for efficient carotenoid extraction (relative content of lipid to carotenoids, types and forms of the carotenoid present, etc.).

In the case of lycopene, the analysis is particularly complex due to low solubility (less soluble in alcohols than α-carotene, β-carotene or xantophylls) and the instability of this compound. Many different extraction procedures have been developed in order to efficiently extract lycopene from food samples. These have included various types of solvent combinations and procedures. Some comparative studies about the relative efficacies of these methods have been performed, including interlaboratory studies, showing that lycopene has the higher variability in carotenoid analysis methods (7).

The most important points that should be taken into account for the analysis of lycopene in foods are: sampling and sample preparation, extraction solvent and extraction procedure.

Sampling and sample preparation

The sampling protocol must consider the variation among different fruits and the different distribution of lycopene in each fruits; usually it is higher in the outer part. Samples should be ground or cut into small pieces to facilitate a complete and homogeneous extraction. Some authors recommend a previous blanching for vegetable tissue containing lipoxygenase (8, 9).

The use of low-moisture samples (< 10 %) usually simplifies the extraction process, and for this reason freeze-drying or desiccation in a vacuum-oven is often carried out to reduce water content in the samples with little damage to the carotenoids. According to some studies (10,11), freeze-drying does not produce significant changes in carotenoids, since it excludes O_2. Long time storage of freeze-drying samples can cause carotenoid alterations, and for this reason freeze-dried samples should be analyzed as soon as possible and stored in a dark place(12). However, some authors do not recommend a complete dehydratation before extractions, since a small amount of water is often useful when a low-polarity solvent mixture is used in the extraction(13, 14).

Sugars can interfere with carotenoids determination when they are present in high amounts; for this reason Wilberg and Rodriguez Amaya (15) recommended their solubilization in a 100 g/L NaCl solution before the carotenoid extraction to avoid this problem with high-sugar containing processed products.

All the materials should be kept away from light (by the use of amber glassware or dimly lit lab areas), atmospheric oxygen, contact with acids and high temperatures (they should be kept at less than 40 °C) to avoid losses of lycopene, and the analysis should be done as rapidly as possible. Some authors also recommended refrigeration conditions for carotenoid extraction (16); Tonucci *et al*. (17) performed the extraction of carotenoids from tomato products at 0 °C under gold fluorescent lights.

Extraction solvent:

Various organic solvents of high purity, or combinations, have been proposed to extract lycopene and other carotenoids from food matrix (Table 1).

REFERENCE	SAMPLES	EXTRACTION
Hart & Scott (1995)50	Vegetables	THF / Methanol (1/1) → Petroleum ether → DCM Saponification: 10 % KOH / Methanol, 1 h RT
Wilberg & Rodriguez Amaya (1995)15	Fruits	Ethanol / Hexane (1/1) Saponification 10 % KOH, 5-10 min
Konings & Roomans (1997)16	Fruits and vegetables	THF / Methanol (1/1) Saponification: KOH 10%, 2 h, RT
Müller (1997)30	Vegetables	Acetone / Ethanol + pyrogalol Saponification 40 % KOH /Methanol
Wright & Kader (1997)49	Fruits	Ethanol / Hexane Saponification: 10 % KOH / Methanol
Ben-Amotz & Fishler (1998)13	Vegetables	THF / Methanol (1/1) → Hexane → DCM
Anguelova & Warthensen (2000)3	Tomato powder	THF / Methanol (50/50) → Petroleum ether → Hexane
Cadoni et al. (2000)33	Tomato	Supercritical CO_2
Otles & Atli (2000)41	Tomato paste	Acetone → Hexane Saponification
Setiawan et al. (2001)25	Fruits	THF → Mobile phase

Table1: Conditions applied by several authors for Lycopene analysis by HPLC

COLUMN	MOBILE PHASE	DETECTION
Guard column ODS2 (Alltech Associates), 22 °C	ACN / Methanol / DCM (75/20/5) + TEA + BHT + Amonium acetate	450 nm
Novapak C18 (Waters)	ACN / CHCl3 (92/8)	436 nm
Vydac 201 TP54 C18 (Vydac)	Methanol / THF (95/5)	DA (450nm)
Vydac C18 (Vydac)	Methanol / Acetone (95/5)	450 nm
Guard column Vydac 201 TP54 C18 (Vydac)	ACN / Methanol / DCM (75/20/5) + BHT + TEA	450 nm
Vydac 201 TP54 C18 (Vydac)	Methanol / ACN (90/10)	450 nm
Vydac 201 TP54 C18 (Vydac)	ACN / Methanol / 2-Propanol (44/54/2)	DA (450 nm)
Spherisorb C18	Methanol / THF / Water (67/27/6)	446 nm
Bondadapack C18 (Waters)	ACN / Methanol (70/30)	450 nm
Ultramex C18 (Phenomenex)	ACN / THF / Methanol + amonium acetate (65 / 25 / 6 / 4)	UV detector

REFERENCE	SAMPLES	EXTRACTION
Craft (2001)24	(1)	Direct dilution in THF + BHT
Craft (2001)24	(2)	Methanol / THF 50/50 + $MgCO_3$ Dilution in alcohol until THF < 10 %
Craft (2001)24	(3)	Saponification : 40 % KOH / Methanol, 60 °C, 1 h Extraction 75/25 hexane/THFDilution in alcohol
Craft (2001)24		
Craft (2001)24		
Granado et al. (2001)27	Vegetables	Hexane / DCM Saponification: KOH 20 %, 3-5 min
Lee & Chen (2001)42	Tomato	Hexane / Acetone / Ethanol (50/25/25) OCC
Niizu & Rodriguez-Amaya (2005)45	Vegetables	Acetone – Petroleum ether
Olives et al. (2006)23	Fruits and vegetables	Hexane / Acetone / Ethanol (50/25/25) →THF / ACN / Methanol (15/30/55)
Raffo et al. (2006)47	Tomato	THF + BHT→ $CHCl_3$ →ACN / Methanol / Hexane / DCM
Sánchez-Moreno et al. (2006)26	Tomato products	THF + BHT→DiethyletHer →DCM → ACN /Methanol/ DCM (45/5/50)

(1) Oil-based food samples with no xantophylls, esters and chlorophylls.
(2) Low lipid samples with no xantophylls, esters and chlorophylls.
(3) Samples containing xantophylls, esters, chlorophyls or high lipid and low carotenoid conte

COLUMN	MOBILE PHASE	DETECTION
Vydac 201 TP or 218 TP C18(Vydac)	Methanol / ACN 90/10 + 0,1 % TEA	450 nm
Vydac 201 TP or 218 TP C18 (Vydac)	Methanol / ACN 90/10 + 0,1 % TEA	450 nm
		450 nm
C30 (Waters)	Gradient: Methanol / Isopropyl alcohol / THF (+ BHT + TEA + Ammonium acetate)	450 nm
Lichrosorb Si (Phenomenex)	Hexane / Dioxane / Indole-3-propionic acid /TEA (80/20/1,5/0,2)	450 nm
Guard column Spher-5-RP-18 (Kontron)	ACN / DCM / Methanol (70/20/10)	450 nm
YMC Carotenoid C30 (YMC)	1-Butanol / ACN / DCM (30/70/10)	DA
Spherisorb S3 ODS2	Gradient: ACN + TEA / Methanol / Ethyl acetate	DA
µBondapack C18 (Waters), 30 °C	Methanol / ACN 90/10 + 0,1 % TEA	475 nm
Supelcosil C18, 30 °C	Gradient: ACN / Methanol / Hexane / DCM	DA (470 nm)
Hypercosil ODS (Technocroma)	Gradient: Hexane / ACN / DCM	DA (470 nm)

DCM = dichloromethane
MTBE= methyl-terc-buthyl-eter
RT = room temperature
DA = Photodiode Array Detector
THF = tetrahydrofuran
BHT = butyl-hydroxy-toluene
ACN = acetonitrile
TEA = triethylamine

Lycopene is not soluble in methanol (a solvent widely used for carotenoids analysis); for this reason, lycopene extraction with a methanol-containing solvent, often requires several extraction steps, with the result of higher volumes and a more complex treatment of the extracts. Solvents commonly used for lycopene extraction are ethanol, hexane, acetone, ethyl acetate, chloroform dichloromethane, isopropanol, petroleum ether (18-20).

Pesek *et al.*(21) reported that chlorinated solvents could induce the formation of 9-*cis* and 13-*cis* isomers of carotenoids; however tetrahydrofurane (THF) or acetonitrile do not have this effect. THF rapidly dissolves carotenoid compounds and denatures proteins, avoiding the formation of emulsions, but it induces peroxide formation, and for this reason an antioxidant agent is often added to this solvent for carotenoid extraction. Also diethylether must be freshly prepared (peroxide-free) before use (8). The use of non-polar solvents such as hexane or tetrahydrofuran (THF) in the extraction solvent makes possible a more efficient extraction and reduces the extraction time and the number of extraction procedures.

These solvents can be applied directly to dry material, but for the extraction from fresh tissues, with a high water content, some water-miscible organic solvents (such as acetone, methanol, ethanol or mixtures) should be added to the extraction medium. In this case, after the extraction, the pigment is transferred from the water-containing extract to the water-immiscible solvent by adding enough water or a saturated NaCl solution until two layers separate (8, 22).

The method recommended by Craft applies methanol / tetrahydrofurane (THF) (50:50 v/v) until the extract is colorless (which usually can take more than 3 or 4 extraction steps in lycopene-rich samples) (24); other authors have used combinations of hexane / acetone / ethanol (50/25/25), with very good results in efficiency of lycopene extraction from foods, with only one extraction step (22, 23).

Antioxidant agents, such as butyl-hydroxide-toluene (BHT), vitamin E, rosemary extract or pyrogallol, are often added to THF to avoid oxidation process during the analytical procedure (23,47). Some neutralizing agents such as alkaline carbonates can also be included in the extraction medium (9, 16, 24) .

Extraction procedure

The lycopene extraction should be repeated several times, until all lycopene has been removed from the sample. Some authors (24, 25) stop the extraction process when the sample is colorless, and other authors (22) repeat the extraction process until no lycopene is found in the extracted sample. Partitioning, washing and phase separation are sometimes applied to the extract, in order to change solvents or eliminate undesirable compounds in the extracts; for example partitioning with petroleum ether and methanol has been used to separate chrolophylls and carotenes in the organic phase and xanthophylls in the alcoholic phase, from tomato seeds (3, 9, 13, 26).

Some extraction solvents can interfere with the High Performance Liquid Chromatography (HPLC) mobile phases used for the separation of carotenoids. They can produce chromatographic artefacts, broaden, or deform the chromatographic peaks. This interaction is usually produced by non-polar extraction solvents (hexane or THF) and more polar HPLC solvents (methanol or acetonitrile)(23). For this reason evaporation (if possible under N_2) is sometimes necessary followed by a redissolution in the mobile phase or in other non-interfering solvents. These practices usually cause a compromise between compatibility with mobile phase and good solubility of lycopene (which can in these cases usually be restricted to 3 - 6 μg/ml maximum) (23, 16).

Saponification is sometimes a necessary step in determination of some carotenoids in plant foods (especially xanthophylls in chlorophyll-rich samples), as it is the optimal method for removal of chlorophylls (which could otherwise sensitize photoisomerization of carotenoids), unwanted lipids (as triglycerides in lipid-rich samples) and other interfering compounds, as well as the best way to hydrolyze carotenoid esters (27, 28). Lycopene, as a hydrocarbon compound, does not form ester linkages and can be directly extracted by homogenizing in the presence of lipophilic solvents, specially in samples with low content of chlorophylls (24), but sometimes a saponification step has been reported to improve accuracy of lycopene analysis in some cases (27).

Although saponification may be carried out directly with the homogenized matrix, it is frequently performed after organic extraction. Different conditions have been used for the saponification: hydrolysis time, temperature, KOH concentration, number and volume for partition and washing (Table 1). Most of them use an alkaline treatment with 10 - 40% KOH / methanol, during 5 - 60 min at 56 - 100 °C or 3 - 16 hours at ambient temperature.

The disadvantage of this treatment is that certain saponification conditions may cause degradation of carotenoids, and for this reason the concentration of KOH, time and temperature must be carefully assessed for the particular type of materials (14). Kimura *et al* (29) performed a thorough study on saponification procedures and effects on foods carotenoids, finding quantitative losses, *trans-cis* isomerization and epoxidation with most of the procedures used (29). These authors recommended saponification at room temperature in petroleum ether with 10% methanolic KOH, either under an N_2 atmosphere or in the presence of an antioxidant, and they state that this procedure is unnecessary for the determination of carotenoids in tomato and kale.

Müller (30) reported the greatest losses for lycopene (about 25 %), compared to other carotenoids in saponifed extracts of vegetables and fruits. He found that the xantophylls were the most resistant. On the contrary, Khachik *et al*. (31) and Scott (2) found greater losses of xantophylls than carotenes after 3 h of saponification at ambient temperature. Short saponification times are desirable to minimize these losses. Wilberg and Rodriguez-Amaya (15) applied 5-10 min saponification with 10 % KOH and Granado *et al*. (27) developed a rapid saponification protocol (40 % KOH/methanol, 5 min), which improved considerably accuracy for lycopene HPLC determination in vegetables, with negligible degree of lycopene isomerization, due to shorter exposure of the sample to alkaline conditions.

For these reasons, saponification is recommended for chlorophyll-rich samples, and the need for this procedure should be assayed depending on the food matrix, the analytical method and the particular interest of the analysis(28). If saponification using alkaline and heat conditions has to be used, BHT should be avoided in the solvents, since in these conditions it can form polymers that absorb light in the visible range and may co-elute with some carotenoids in HPLC analysis(24) .

In order to know the magnitude of possible losses of carotenoids during the analytical procedures, internal standards as ethyl-β-apo-8'-carotenoate, echinenone or retinil palmitate, are sometimes added to samples (13, 16, 32) .

Another way to extract carotenoids in food samples is supercritical fluid extraction. This is an advanced separation technique based on the enhanced solvating power of gases above their critical point. The preferred gas is CO_2, because it has a low critical temperature and it is non-toxic, non-flammable and low cost and high purity. It can be used at temperatures of 40-80 °C and pressures of 35 –70 MPa. Supercritical fluid extraction has been suggested as an alternative method for selective isolation of carotenoids in one step, avoiding the use of organic solvents or elevated processing temperatures. Supercritical fluid extraction can be compatible with supercritical fluid chromatography since the two techniques can share the mobile phase and same devices, favouring the development of extraction and separation methodologies. This technique has been applied to successfully separate lycopene from other carotenoids in tomato fruits (5, 33-36).

IDENTIFICATION AND QUANTIFICATION

Carotenoid analysis in food products may be done by different methods: HPLC, spectrophotometry, or by the evaluation of the colour (5). Although spectrophotometry or colorimetry can be used to rapidly assess the lycopene content of products derived from tomatoes, a highly versatile, sensitive and selective method such as HPLC is needed for reliable analysis of food samples. The election of the analytical method depends on the particular interest of the analysis and the kind of product analyzed.

Spectrophotometric methods

Spectrophotometric methods are simple, but lack specificity for carotenoid analysis. However, they have been shown to be reliable methods for identifying lycopene as the major pigment present in a mixture. The differences in absorption spectrum between lycopene and other major carotenoids in foods such as β-carotene, α-carotene or lutein make the quantification of lycopene at its characteristic maximum of 503nm easy, with no interference of other compounds, in lycopene-rich samples such as tomato or watermelon. Fish *et al.* (37) stated that in samples where lycopene is at least 70 % of the constituent carotenoids, the contribution of carotenoids other than lycopene to absorbance at 503 nm is less than 2 % for watermelon, 4 % for tomato and 6 % for pink grapefruit.

A wide number of lycopene studies have been published using this method (22,38, 39), as it allows quick routine analysis in the above-mentioned samples. Fish *et al.* (37) have also reported a spectrophotometric method with the advantage of using reduced volumes of organic solvents. For quantification purposes, the molar extinction coefficient lycopene can be used (40), avoiding problems of instability and availability of commercial standards.

Chromatographic methods

Chromatographic methods are specific and allow the separation of different compounds. However, Gas Chromatography is not suitable for carotenoid analysis, since these compounds decompose when exposed to the high temperatures use by this technique.

From all the possible Liquid Chromatography methods for lycopene analysis, Open Column Chromatography (OCC) has been used especially for preparative purposes, with absorbents such as alumina or silica gel, MgO, $CaCO_3$, sugar or cellulose, and eluents of increasing polarity (starting with hexane) to obtain different fractions of pigments depending on the polarity. These fractions can be then analyzed by spectrophotometry(9).

To improve the slow rate, diatomaceous earth can be mixed with the absorbent in various proportions (8). Otles and Atli (41) used a MgO-silica gel column, with a top layer of anhydrous Na_2SO_4 to analyze carotenoids from tomato paste and compared it with HPLC, obtaining comparable results between both methods. OCC has the advantage of being more economical to perform but is more time consuming.

Thin Layer Chromatography (TLC) has been successfully applied for carotenoid separation and purification from tomato, either alone or in combination with OCC. By OCC the carotenoids can be first separated into fractions of different polarity, which are then further separated into individual compounds by TLC, using MgO, diatomaceous earth and cellulose as the absorbent, and with solvent systems consisting of hexane, isopropanol and methanol (8). A chromato-scanner can be used as the detection system or a High Performance TLC (HPTLC) system can be applied to accurately quantify the compounds detected.

Numerous papers have been published on the HPLC analysis of carotenoids including lycopene from food samples. These techniques permit the separation, identification and quantification of different carotenoid compounds separately, and even distinguish between geometrical structures of carotenoids, including some mono- and *di-cis*-isomers (42, 43) .

Stewart and Wheaton (44) developed the first HPLC method applied to carotenoid analysis, which was normal-phase using a laboratory-packed MgO column with a linear gradient of hexane / acetone containing 10 % benzene. This method could separate several carotenoids in tomato samples, including lycopene. After this, several methods have been carried out to analyze lycopene in food matrix by HPLC, especially reverse-phase (RP) ones.

Several RP-HPLC columns are suitable for HPLC analysis of lycopene in food samples (Table 1). Niizu *et al.* (45) used a monomeric C18 column to achieve carotenoid separation from salad vegetables; however, Jinno and Lin (46) recommended the use of polymeric ODS stationary phase, for its better selectivity than monomeric ODS columns, taking into account their molecular shape and size recognition, as well as the better separation obtained with them. Most authors use C18 RP-columns for lycopene analysis (27, 30, 47), as they can provide good resolution for lycopene and other carotenoids. The use of metal free columns and frits (such as titanium ones) is desirable, to avoid damage to the carotenoids during the analysis (2).

C30 RP-columns were specifically developed for the separation of carotenoids(48). This stationary phase, with a very high efficiency, is preferred when the interest is focused on the separation of different isomers of carotenoids, including the positional and geometrical ones. Yeum *et al.* (43) separated 5 isomers of lycopene by using a C30 column and a gradient solvent system of methanol / methyl-*terc*-butyl-eter (MTBE) / water. Lee and Chen (42) compared two types of column (C18 and C30) and various solvent systems for separation. All-*trans*-lycopene and 9 *cis* isomers (5-*cis*, 9-*cis*, 13-*cis*, 15-*cis* and 4 di-*cis*-lycopene) were resolved by employing a C30 column with a mobile phase of n-butanol-acetonitrile-dichloromethane (30:70:10, v/v/v) within 35 min.

A guard column with a stationary phase similar to the column is sometimes used to increase the life of the column and improve the resolution of the peaks (27, 49, 50). The control of column temperature is an additional important factor in reducing analytical variation of the results, especially with C30 stationary phases (51), and it can be also useful to speed up the analysis. Temperatures should not be higher than 30 °C (to avoid isomerization); however, the effect of temperature should be assessed for each system, and conditions should be optimized for each case (46, 52).

Regarding to the mobile phases (Table 1), they may include solvents such as acetonitrile, methanol, 1-butanol, 2-propanol, ethyl acetate, THF, water, MTBE, or halogenated hydrocarbons (such as dichloromethane or chloroform). Despite the poor solubility of lycopene in methanol, this solvent can be included in some proportion in the mobile phase, taking into account that all the solutions injected should not have a high concentration of lycopene to avoid precipitation in the column or frits (24). The use of gradients is sometimes applied to achieve a better separation of the compounds.

The addition of a solvent modifier such as *n*-decanol, N,N-diisopropyl-ethylamine or triethylamine (TEA) to the mobile phase, in quantities ranging between 0,05-0,1 %, has been shown to prevent non-specific absorption and oxidation, and thus, improve recovery of carotenoids; it also may reduce retention times with no compromise of resolution (24, 50). A mobile phase consisting of 90 / 10 methanol / acetonitrile and 0,1 % TEA has shown goods results in lycopene separation from other carotenoids in several food samples (23, 24).

The most simple HPLC detection system for lycopene is UV-visible; usually λ of 475 nm is used, because it allows the quantification of other carotenoids present in the sample. A photodiode array detector is useful to identify and quantify lycopene and other carotenoids in food samples, following simultaneously the elution on the full UV-visible range, which guarantee that each pigment can be identified by its spectrum and quantified at its absorbance maximum.

Olives *et al*. (23), optimized and compared an HPLC method with the spectrophotometric standard method mentioned above, for the determination of lycopene and ß-carotene in vegetables. They used extraction on different fruits and vegetables with hexane/acetone/ethanol (50:25:25 v/v/v), evaporation of hexane layer, redissolution in THF/ACN/methanol (15:30:55 v/v/v) and injection on a C18 column with methanol/ACN (90:10 v/v) + TEA 9 µM, as mobile phase (a flow rate of 0.9 ml/min) and detection at 475 nm. The HPLC method was comparable to the standard spectrophotometric method in precision, accuracy and sensitivity, with a simple preparation of the samples (one step direct extraction) and short run times (10 min) for the quantification of lycopene in fruit and vegetable samples.

Other detection systems include a coulometric electrochemical detector, recommended when very low levels of carotenoids need to be quantified (24, 53), or Mass Spectrometry (MS) which should be performed under a temperature of 100°C, due to heat instability of carotenoids. MS allows the identification of lycopene and other carotenoids based on the structural information obtained from the fragmentation of the molecules provided by classical ionization methods (such as electron impact and chemical ionization), or by soft ionization techniques (as fast atom bombardment, matrix-assisted laser desorption / ionization, electrospray ionization and atmospheric pressure chemical ionization), which have facilitated the molecular weight determination of carotenoids by minimizing fragmentation. The differentiation of structural isomers (such as carotene and lycopene) can be carried out with the aid of collision-induced dissociation and tandem mass spectrometry, which augment fragmentation and obtain structurally significant fragment ions. For example, the ion of $[M\text{-}69]^{+*}$, indicating the presence of a terminal acyclic isoprene unit, is observed in the tandem mass spectra of lycopene, neurosporene and γ-carotene, but not for α-carotene, β-carotene, lutein or zeaxantine (54).

However, the structural elucidation of carotenoid stereoisomers can only be accomplished by the use of nuclear magnetic resonance spectroscopy (NMR). HPLC-NMR on-line coupling has been shown to be particularly advantageous since it allows the direct identification of carotenoid stereosiomers in food as well as in physiological samples(55).

Calibration of detection HPLC equipment with pure standards is often necessary, although standards for many carotenoids are unavailable commercially. The accuracy of the results would depend on the purity of these standards. In the case of lycopene, commercial standards of all-*trans*-lycopene can be used for identification and quantification purposes. *Cis*-lycopene can be tentatively identified based on their spectral properties: they have smaller extinction coefficients than the all-*trans* form; the mono-*cis* isomers result in a hypsocromic shift of about 4 nm when compared to the all-*trans* form; the central *cis*-isomers have a strong peak at about 340 nm and the di-*cis* isomers may be shifted to shorter wavelength than its mono-*cis* isomers (42, 56-58) .

The use of commercial standards has the disadvantage of being expensive and unstable. For this reason, they should be verified using a spectrophotometer to avoid errors in quantification due to possible impurities and to the fact that carotenoids dissolve slowly in many solvents. Accuracy of the analysis can be improved by calculating the real concentration of the standard solution from the absorbance and the extinction coefficient. The value assigned can be further refined by correcting for peak purity, which is obtained from the spectrum of each standard. Once the standard solution concentrations have been established, the individual standard solution can be mixed to form the final calibration solutions(24).

All the standards should be daily prepared, used immediately and the use of stock solutions is not desirable, due to degradation risk. Although lycopene solutions can be stable for one week at –20 °C if protected from light and oxygen(24), if standard stock solutions are to be used, they should be daily evaluated for purity by the measurements of absorbance or chromatographic peak area (16). The precipitation of lycopene can also take place in standard solutions when placed at freeze temperatures; in this case, the standard must be redissolved by agitation in an ultrasonic bath, or filtered to reassign its concentration.

Due to the problems of availability and instability of commercial standards of lycopene, some authors prefer to prepare their own standards by means of extraction from tomato samples, purification and evaluation of the concentration. For this purpose the usual organic solvent used for carotenoid extraction can be used, followed by concentration in a rotatory evaporator. OCC has been also used for purification purposes in a MgO:Hyflosupercel column (45). Rodriguez (14) also recommended the purification of carotenoids using crystallization of fractions derived from a preparatory chromatographic technique such as TLC or OCC.

Interlaboratory studies on HPLC procedures for carotenoids analysis on foods have shown relative uncertainties attributed to the effect of the chromatographic system and standardization of carotenoid extract, whereas the preparation of the carotenoid extract (protocol and efficiency) may account for more than half of the total variance (7,59). To evaluate the magnitude of these uncertainties, some certificate standard reference materials (CRM), available from different institutions, can be used(27), which are essential to the development and harmonization of methods. Scott *et al*. (7) developed a CRM consisting of a mixture of freeze-dried vegetables, including tomato, which kept a 97 % retention after 36 months stored at −18 °C under nitrogen and out of the incidence of light. There are some commercially available CRM for carotenoid analysis, consisting of vegetable mixtures and baby food composite; however, lycopene content of these materials is usually given not as a certified value but as a reference one, due to the instability of this pigment.

Other methods

Other estimation methods have been performed in lycopene-rich fruits such as tomato and tomato products, using spectroscopic measurements.

The characteristic red color of tomato fruits results from a combination of carotenoid pigments, of which lycopene is the most abundant. Polder *et al*. (60) investigated the surface distribution of carotenes and chlorophyll on tomatoes at different stages of ripening, using imaging spectroscopy. Spectral images were obtained within the range 400-700 nm (with a resolution of 1 nm), and samples were also analyzed by HPLC for chlorophylls and carotenoids analysis. These authors found significant correlations between spectral images and HPLC data of pigments including lycopene, concluding that such methods could be used to sort tomatoes according to concentration and uniformity of distribution of these compounds.

Davis *et al*.(38), used a scanning xenon flash colorimeter spectrophotometer to directly measure light absorbance on tomato puree, which correlated to lycopene content of the samples. Other authors, such as D'Souza *et al* (61), have used tristimulus colorimeters to measure reflected visible color or to read the fruit chromaticity, based on the CIE ("Commision Internationale de L'Eclairage") color space coordinates L* (degree of lightness or value), a* (a measure of the degree of redness or greenness) and b* (a measure of the degree of yellowness or blueness). From these parameters, the color hue values, the relations, the saturation and chroma values are calculated to show the relationship among colors. Hue and chroma value are elements studied to characterize the viewing colors three dimensionally.

These parameters have been correlated to lycopene content in tomato products, better than surface reflectance readings(62). Fernandez *et al*. (63) obtained high correlations of results using different equipment, and a* value of tomato juice was shown as a good predictor for lycopene content in tomato juice. These methods are inexpensive and reliable, don't require hazardous chemicals, and for this reason, although sometimes they do not entirely substitute for the chemical extraction analysis, they are useful for estimating lycopene concentration for routine analysis required by breeders, producers and researchers.

Other methods, based on reflected and scattered light have been used to estimate pigment content and to predict color of vegetables. Nowadays great interest is focused on the use of non-destructive rapid techniques for food components analysis. These methods are being evaluated for non-volatile compounds analysis in vegetables (including lycopene), using laser technology coupled with Mass Spectrometry, having the advantage of no need for the extraction procedures necessary for spectrophotometric or chromatographic methods.

MEASUREMENT OF ANTIOXIDANT ACTIVITY OF LYCOPENE IN FOOD SAMPLES

Carotenoids, vitamins C and E, and phenolic compounds are the most naturally occurring plant substances with antioxidant activity. Lycopene, a carotenoid and lipophilic antioxidant, plays a crucial role in biological systems by providing protection against cardiovascular disease and some cancers and by boosting the immune system as it quenches highly reactive singlet oxygen ($O_2^{\bullet -}$) and traps peroxiradicals ($ROO^{\bullet}$)(64). Several studies (47,65-68) have investigated the effects of ripening stage, genotype and processing on the hydrophilic and lipophilic antioxidant activity of tomato by using different analysis methods for antioxidant activity measurements. Generally, hydrophilic antioxidant activity is significantly affected by genotype and processing, and almost independent of the ripening stage; on the other hand, lipophilic antioxidant activity is more influenced by ripening stage than by genotype.

The evaluation of fruit antioxidant capacity is not a simple task. Many methods have been proposed for this determination. They vary in their use of substrates, conditions, analytical methods, and concentrations; each may affect the estimated activity (69).

Most of the methods for the total antioxidant activity (TAA) are generally based on the inhibition of certain reactions by the presence of antioxidants. Many of these are based on the removal of generated free radicals by the presence of antioxidants. These includes the trolox equivalent antioxidant capacity (TEAC) method, the 2,2-azinobis-3-ethylbenzothiazoline-6-sulphonate (ABTS) method, the total radical-trapping antioxidant (TRAP) method, the 2,2-diphenyl-1-picrylhydrazl (DPPH) method, and the N,N-dimethyl-p-phenylenediamine (DMPD) method, to name just a few (70,71).

Methods based on the evaluation of the free radical scavenging capacity of a food

Free radical scavenging activity (RSA) of food samples can be measured with different reagents such as: 1,1-diphenyl-2-picrylhydrazyl radical ($DPPH^{\bullet}$) ; 2,2'-azinobis(3-ethylbenzo-thiazo-line-6-sulfonate) ($ABTS^{\bullet+}$) or DMDP. A commercially available free radical, which is soluble in methanol, is ($DPPH^{\bullet+}$) (2,2 diphenyl-1-picrylhydrazyl) (72). With this free radical, the antioxidant activity of a food is measured by mixing with this free radical and following the decrease in absorbance at 515 nm until a steady state is reached. The activity is measured at ambient temperature to eliminate the risk of thermal degradation of the analyzed compounds. Depending on the antioxidant, the neutralization kinetics can take from minutes to six hours or more (72). This method was applied by Sánchez-Moreno *et al.* (26) after tomato puree was subjected to high pressure or traditional thermal processing. Their results indicated that samples treated with high pressure showed a higher carotenoid content with no loss of antioxidant activity.

$ABTS^{\bullet+}$ is generated enzymatically by addition of H_2O_2 and peroxidase, which is a coloured free radical, whose neutralization is followed by reading the decrease in absorbance at 400-750 nm after the addition of the antioxidant (73). In this method the antioxidant activity is related to Trolox (a water soluble analogue of vitamin E) and expressed as mmol of Trolox per gram of food sample (TEAC, Trolox equivalent antioxidant activity). This method with slight modifications was applied by Arnao *et al* (74) to study the hydrophilic and lipophilic contribution total antioxidant activity. Sahlin *et al.* (75) evaluated the antioxidant properties of tomatoes after processing using the modified $ABTS^{+}$ method. Results indicated that cooking had a deleterious effect on these properties and frying caused the largest loss of antioxidant compounds and antioxidant activity. Toor *et al.* (39) evaluated the seasonal variations in antioxidants composition of tomato fruit and found that lycopene content was lower in summer months, which was mainly due by the higher temperatures (above 30°C). These results were confirmed by Raffo *et al.* (47) who reported that greenhouse-growing conditions of tomato fruit induced an accumulation of carotenoids for most of the year.

DMPD (N, N-dimethyl-p-phenylene diamine dihydrochloride) Method. This assay is based on the reduction of buffered solution of colored DMPD in acetate buffer and ferric chloride. The colored free radical cation ($DMPD^{\bullet+}$) is generated by addition of Fe^{3+} to *p*-phenylene diamine, and its disappearance is followed by measuring the absorbance at 505 nm (76).

The oxygen radical absorbance capacity assay (ORAC assay) determines free radical scavenging activity against the peroxyl radical for both water-soluble and lipid-soluble substances. The scavenging capacity of antioxidants in nutrients or *in vivo* against the peroxyl radical, which is one of the most common reactive oxygen species (ROS) found in the body, is measured. The ORAC-hydro assay reflects water-soluble antioxidant capacity, while the ORAC-lipo assay measures lipid-soluble antioxidant capacity. The values of these two assays are additive. Trolox, a water-soluble vitamin E analog, is used as the calibration standard and the ORAC result is expressed as micromole Trolox equivalent (TE) per gram. Even though the ORAC assays do not measure the scavenging capacity against a large body of free radicals, it is a valid and meaningful representation of antioxidant capacity (77,78). Dávalos (79) has introduced a modification of the method which is called ORAC-fluoresceine (ORAC-FL). Bangalore *et al* (80) validated the ORAC assay for various concentrations of lycopene in the presence of beta-cyclodextrin, a water-solubility enhancer.

The antioxidant capacity can also be determined in plasma by the total antioxidant capacity test (TAC) (81-83). TAC is based on the capacity of antioxidants in plasma to diminish the oxidation of an added substrate (crocine) under defined conditions. TAC of an antioxidant is determined at 37° C, in a plasma with a pH of 7,4. 2,2' azo-bis-(2 metilpropionamide) dihidrocloro (AAPH) is used to generate the free radicals (R°, RO°, ROO°) that will oxidize the crocine. The crocine concentration is followed by measuring the absorbance at 439 nm.

Total radical-trapping antioxidant parameter assay (TRAP assay) is another method. Its precision has been questioned (77), because the oxygen electrode may not remain stable during the measurement period.

Methods based on measuring the iron-reducing capacity (FRAP) of food samples

The FRAP method measures the ferric reducing ability in plasma at a low pH (84). An intense blue colour is formed when the ferric-tripyridyltriazine (Fe^{3+}-TPTZ) complex is reduced to the ferrous (Fe^{2+}). There is a linear correlation with the absorption at 593 nm and the total reducing capacity of the antioxidants donors of electrons. In the FRAP method the activity is related to ascorbic acid (vitamin C) and expressed as mmol ascorbic acid per gram of food sample (AEAC, ascorbic acid equivalent antioxidant activity).

The antioxidant activity of fresh tomatoes and tomato paste was investigated by Takeoka *et al*. with this assay (85). Three fractions (i.e. aqueous, methanol, and hexane fractions) were obtained from the fresh tomatoes and paste. A free radical quenching assay and a singlet oxygen quenching assay, found significant antioxidant activity in both the hexane fraction (containing lycopene) and the methanol fraction, (containing the phenolic antioxidants caffeic and chlorogenic acid). The results from these authors suggested that in addition to lycopene, polyphenols in tomatoes may also be important in conferring protective antioxidative effects.

REFERENCES:

1. Rodriguez-Amaya DB. A guide to carotenoid analysis in foods. Washington, DC, USA: ILSI Press 1999.
2. Scott KJ. Observations on some of the problems associated with the analysis of carotenoids in foods by HPLC. Food Chem 1992; 45: 357-364.
3. Anguelova T, Warthesen J. Lycopene stability in tomato powders. J Food Sci 2000; 65(1): 67-70.
4. Shi J, Maguer M, Bryan M, Kakuda Y. Kinetics of lycopene degradation in tomato puree by heat and light irradiation. J Food Process Eng 2003; 25(6): 485-498.
5. Schoefs B. Chlorophyll and carotenoid analysis in food products. Properties of the pigments and methods of analysis. Trends Food Sci Technol 2002; 13: 361- 371.
6. Bicanic D, Anese M, Luterotti S, Dadarlat D, Gibkes J. Lubbers M. Rapid, accurate and direct determination of total lycopene content in tomato paste. Review of Scientific Instruments 2003; 74 (1) Part 2: 687-689.
7. Scott KJ, Finglas PM, Seale R, Hart DJ, de Froidmont-Görtz I. Interlaboratory studies of HPLC procedures for the analysis of carotenoids in foods. Food Chem 1996; 57: 85-90.
8. Gross J. Pigments in vegetables. New York, USA: Van Nostrand Reinhold 1991.
9. AOAC (Association of Official Analitical Chemists). Official Methods of Analysis. Herlich K (ed.) Arlington, USA 1990.
10. Desobry SA, Netto FM, Labuza TP. Preservation of β-carotene from carrots. Crit. Rev. Food Sci. Nutr 1998; 38 (5): 381-397.
11. González Castro MJ, Oruña Concha MJ, Lopez Hernandez J, Simal Lozano J. Effect of freeze-drying on the composition of green beans and Padrón peppers. Deut Lebensm Runds 1998; 94 (1): 89-91.
12. Ball GFM. Bioavailability and analysis of vitamins in foods. London, England: Chapman and Hall. 1998.
13. Ben-Amotz A, Fishler R. Analysis of carotenoids with emphasis on 9-cis beta-carotene in vegetables and fruits commonly consumed in Israel. Food Chem 1998; 62(4): 515-520.
14. Rodriguez GA Extaction, Isolation, and Purification of Carotenoids. In: Wrolstad R, Acree TE, An H, Decker EA, Penner MH, Reid DS, Schwartz SJ, Shoemaker CF, Sporns P. Current Protocols in Food Analytical Chemistry. New York, USA: John Wiley & Sons 2001: F 2.1.1 — F 2.1.8

15. Wilberg VC, Rodriguez-Amaya DB. HPLC quantitation of major carotenoids of fresh and processed guava, mango and papaya. Lebensmittel Wissenschaft und Technologie. 1995; 28(5): 474-480.
16. Konings EJM, Roomans HHS Evaluation and validation of an LC method for the analysis of carotenoids in vegetables and fruit. Food Chem 1997; 59(4), 599-603.
17. Tonucci LH, Holden JM, Beecher GR, Khachik F, Davis CS, Mulokozi G. Carotenoid content of termally processed tomato-based food products. J Agric Food Chem 1995; 43(3): 579-586.
18. Taungbodhitham AK, Jones GP, Wahlqvist ML, Briggs DR. Evaluation of extraction method for the analysis of carotenoids in fruits and vegetables. Food Chem 1998; 63(4): 577-584.
19. Pichini S, Zuccaro P, Pellegrini M, Di Carlo S, Bacosi A, Palmi I, Tossini G, Pacifici R. . J Liq Chromatogr Relat Technol 2002; 25: 781-786.
20. Lin CH, Chen BH. Determination of carotenoids in tomato juice by liquid chromatography. J Chromat A 2003; 1012: 103.
21. Pesek CA, Warthensen JJ, Taoukis PS. A kinetic model for equilibration of isomeric -carotenes. J Agric Food Chem 1990; 38: 41-45.
22. Sadler G, Davis J, Dezman D. Rapid extraction of lycopene and b-carotene from reconstitued tomato paste and pink grapefruit homogenates. J Food Sci 1990; 55 (5): 1460-1461.
23. Olives Barba AI, Camara Hurtado M, Sanchez Mata MC, Fernandez Ruiz V, Lopez Saenz de Tejada M. Application of a UV-vis detection-HPLC method for a rapid determination of lycopene and beta-carotene in vegetables. Food Chem 2006; 95(2): 328-336.
24. Craft NE. Chromatographic Techniques for Carotenoid Separation. In: Wrolstad R, Acree TE, An H, Decker EA, Penner MH, Reid DS, Schwartz SJ, Shoemaker CF, Sporns P. Current Protocols in Food Analytical Chemistry. New York, USA: John Wiley & Sons 2001: F2.3.1 — F2.3.15.
25. Setiawan B, Sulaeman A, Giraud DW, Driskell JA. Carotenoid content of selected Indonesian fruits. J Food Comp Anal 2001; 14(2): 169-176 .
26. Sánchez-Moreno C, Plaza L, De Ancos B, Cano P. Impact of hich-pressure and traditional thermal processing of tomato purée on carotenoids, vitamin C and antioxidant activity. J Sci Food Agric 2006; 86: 171-179.
27. Granado F, Olmedilla B, Gil Martinez E, Blanco I. A fast, reliable and low-cost saponification protocol for analysis of carotenoids in vegetables. J Food Compos Anal 2001; 14(5): 479-489.
28. Goodwin TW, Britton G. Distribution and analysis of carotenoids. In: T.W. Goodwin. Plant Pigments. London, England: Academic Press. 1988.
29. Kimura M, Rodriguez-Amaya DB, Godoy HT. Assessment of the saponification step in the quantitative determination of carotenoids and provitamins A. Food Chem 1990; 35(3): 187-195.
30. Müller H. Determination of the carotenoid content in selected vegetables and fruit by HPLC and photodiode array detection. Z Lebensm Unters Forsch 1997; 204: 88-94.
31. Khachik F, Beecher GR, Whittaker NF. Separation, identification, and quantification of the major carotenoid and chlorophyll constituents in extracts of several green vegetables by liquid chromatography. J Agric Food Chem 1986; 34: 603-616.
32. Granado F, Olmedilla B, Blanco I, Rojas-Hidalgo E. Carotenoid composition in raw and cooked Spanish vegetables. J Agric Food Chem 1992; 40: 2135-2140.
33. Cadoni EM, De Giorgi R, Medda E, Poma G. Supercritical CO2 extraction of lycopene and β-carotene from ripe tomatoes. Dyes and Pigments 2000; 44: 27-32.

34. Ibañez E, Lopez Sebastian S, Tabera J, Reglero G. Separation of carotenoids by supercritical fluid chromatography with coated, packed capillary columns and neat carbon dioxide. J Chromatogr 1998; 823A: 313-319.
35. Rozzi NL, Singh RK, Vierling RA, Watkins BA. Supercritical fluid extraction of lycopene from tomato processong byproducts. J Agric Food Chem 2002; 50: 2638-2643.
36. Gomez-Prieto MS, Caja MM, Herraiz M, Santa Maria G. Supercritical fluid extraction of all-trans-lycopene from tomato. J Agric Food Chem 2003; 51 (1): 3-7.
37. Fish WW, Perkins-Veazie P, Collins JK. A quantitative assay for lycopene that utilizes reduced volumes of organic solvents. J Food Compos Anal 2002; 15: 309-317.
38. Davis AR, Fish WW, Perkins-Veazie P. A rapid spectrophotometric method for analyzing lycopene content in tomato and tomato products. Postharvest Biol Technol 2003; 28: 425-430.
39. Toor RK, Savage GP, Heeb A. Influence of different types of fertilisers on the major antioxidant components of tomatoes. J Food Compos Anal 2006; 19(1): 20-27.
40. Zechmeister L, LeRosen AL, Schroeder WA, Polgár A, Pauling L. Spectral characteristics and configuration of some stereoisomeric carotenoids including prolycopene and pro-γ carotene. J Amer Chem Soc 1943; 65 (October): 1940-1950.
41. Otles S, Atli Y. Analysis of carotenoids in tomato paste by HPLC and OCC. Am Lab 2000; 32(15): 22-24.
42. Lee MT, Chen BH. Separation of lycopene and its cis isomers by liquid chromatography. Chromatographia 2001; 54(9/10): 613-617.
43. Yeum KJ, Booth SL, Sadowski JA, Liu C, Tang G, Krinsky NI, Russel RM. Human plasma carotenoid response to the ingestion of controlled diets high in fruits and vegetables. Am J Clin Nutr 1996; 64(4): 594-602.
44. Stewart I, Wheaton TA. Continuous flow separation of carotenoids by liquid chromatography J Chrom 1971; 55: 325-336.
45. Niizu PY, Rodriguez Amaya DB. New data on the carotenoid composition of raw salad vegetables. J Food Comp Anal 2005; 18(8): 739-749.
46. Jinno J, Lin Y. Separation of carotenoids by high-performance liquid chromatography with polymeric and monomeric octadecylsilica stationary phases. Chromatographia 1995; 41(5/6): 311-317.
47. Raffo A, Malfa G.la, FoglianoV, Maiani G, Quaglia G.Seasonal variations in antioxidant components of cherry tomatoes (Lycopersicon esculentum cv. Naomi F1). J Food Comp Anal 2006; 19(1): 11-19.
48. Sander LC, Sharpless KE, Craft NE, Wise SA. Development of engineered stationary phases for separation of carotenoid isomers. Anal Chem 1994; 66: 1667-1674.
49. Wright KP, Kader AA. Effect of controlled atmosphere storage on the quality and carotenoid content of sliced persimmons and peaches. Postharvest Biol Technol 1997; 10: 89-97.
50. Hart DJ, Scott J. Development and evaluation of an HPLC method for the analysis of carotenoids in foods, and the measurement of the carotenoid content of vegetables and fruits commonly consumed in the UK. Food Chem 1995; 54: 101-111.
51. Böhm V. Use of column temperature to optimize carotenoid isomer separation by C30 high performance liquid chromatopgraphy. J Sep Sci 2001; 24: 955-959.
52. Scott KJ, Hart DJ. Further observations on problems associated with the analysis of carotenoids by HPLC-2: Column temperature. Food Chem 1993; 47: 403-405.
53. Ferruzzi MG, Sander LC, Rock CL, Schwartz SJ. Carotenoid determination in biological microsamples using liqud chromatography with a coulometric electrochemical array detector. Anal Biochem 1998; 256: 74-81.

54. Van Breemen RB Mass Spectrometry of carotenids. In: Wrolstad R, Acree TE, An H, Decker EA, Penner MH, Reid DS, Schwartz SJ, Shoemaker CF, Sporns P. Current Protocols in Food Analytical Chemistry. New York, USA: John Wiley & Sons 2001: F2.4.1 – F2.4.13.
55. Glaser T, Lienau A, Zeeb D, Krucker M, Dachtler M, Albert K. Qualitative and quantitative determination of carotenoid stereoisomers in a variety of spinach samples by use of MSPD before HPLC-UV, HPLC-APCI-MS, and HPLC-NMR on-line coupling. Chromatographia 2003 Supplement 57: S-9-S-25.
56. Goodwin TW. The biochemistry of carotenoids. Vol. I: Plants. New York, USA: Chapman and Hall 1981.
57. Zechmeister L, Polgár A. Cis-trans isomerization and cis-peak effect in the alpha-carotene set and in some other stereoisomeric sets. J Amer Chem Soc 1944; 66: 137-144.
58. Davies BH. Carotenoids, In: Goodwin TW (ed.). Chemistry and Biochemistry of Plant Pigments Vol. 2. New York, USA: Academic Press 1976: 38-165.
59. Sharpless KE, Arce Osuna M, Brown Thomas J, Gill LM. Value assignment of retinol, retinyl palmitate, tocopherol, and carotenoid concentrations in Standard Reference Material 2383 (Baby Food Composite). J AOAC Int 1999; 82(2): 288-296.
60. Polder G, Heijden GWAM, Voet H, Young IT. Measuring surface distribution of carotenes and chlorophyll in ripening tomatoes using imaging spectrometry. Postharvest Biology and Technology. 2004; 34(2): 117-129.
61. D'Souza MC, Singha S, Ingle M. Lycopene as the most efficient biological carotenoid singlet oxygen quencher. Arch Biochem Biophys 1992; 274: 532-538.
62. Thompson KA, Marshall MR, Sims CA, Wei CI, Sargent SA, Scott JW. Cultivar, maturity and heat treatment on lycopene content in tomatoes. J Food Sci 2000; 65: 791-795.
63. Fernández Ruiz, V.; Cámara, M.; Shoemaker, C. Color and lycopene concentration of fresh market tomatoes and tomato juice. 8th ISHS Symposium on Processing Tomato. Estambul, Turquía 2002.
64. Shi J, Le Maguer M. Lycopene in tomatoes: chemical and physical propoerties affected by food processing. Crit Rev Biotechnol 2000; 20(4): 293-334.
65. Cano A, Acosta M, Arnao M. Hydrophilic and lipophilic antioxidant activity changes during on-vine ripening of tomatoes (Lycopersicon esculentum Mill.). Postharvest Biology and Technology 2003; 28: 59–65.
66. George B, Kaur C, Khurdiya DS, Kapoor H.C, Antioxidants in tomato (Lycopersicon esculentum) as a function of genotype. Food Chemistry 2004; 84: 45–51.
67. Lavelli V, Peri C, Rizzolo A, Antioxidant activity of tomato products as studied by model reactions using xanthine oxidase, myeloperoxidase, and copper-induced lipid peroxidation. Journal of Agricultural and Food Chemistry 2000 ; 48: 1442–1448.
68. Leonardi C, Ambrosino P, Esposito F, Fogliano V. Antioxidative activity and carotenoid and tomatine contents in different typologies of fresh consumption tomatoes. Journal of Agricultural and Food Chemistry 2000. 48: 4723–4727.
69. Frankel EN, Meyer AS. The problems of using one-dimensional methods to evaluate multifunctional food and biological antioxidants. J Sci Food Agric 2000; 80: 1925.
70. Arnao MB, Cano A, Acosta M. Methods to measure the antioxidant activity in plant material. A comparative discussion. 1999 Dec. 31 Suppl:S89-96.
71. Muñoz B. Actividad antirradicalaria en ajo, cebolla y perejil. Memoria DEA. UCM. Madrid, España.

72. Brand-Williams W, Cuvelier ME, Berset C. Use of free radical method to evaluate antioxidant activity. Food Sci. Technol. (London) 1995; 28: 25.
73. Cano A, Hernández-Ruiz J, Garcıán F, Acosta M, Arnao MB. An end-point method for estimation of the total antioxidant activity in plant material. Phytochem Anal 1998; 9: 196.
74. Arnao MB, Cano A, Acosta M. The hydrophilic and lipophilic contribution to total antioxidant acitivity. Food Chem 2001; 73: 239-244.
75. Sahlin E, Savage GP, Lister CE. Investigation of the antioxidant properties of tomatoes after processing. J Food Compos Anal 2005; 17(5): 635-647.
76. Arnao MB, Cano A, Acosta M.Method for measuring antioxidant activity and its application to monitoring the antioxidant capacity of wines.1999 Mar;47(3):1035-40.
77. Prior R, Cao, Guohua. Análisis of botanicals and dietary supplements for antioxidant capacity: a review. Journal of AOAC International. 2000; 83 (4):950-956.
78. Ou B, Hampsch-Woodill M, Prior RL. Development and Validation of Oxygen Radical Absorbance Activity using Fluorescein as the Fluorescent Probe. Journal of Agricultural and Food Chemistry 2001;49:4619-4626.
79. Dávalos A, Gómez-Cordovés C, Bartolomé B. Comercial dietary antioxidant supplements assayed for their antioxidant activity by different methodologies. J Agric Food Chem 2003; 51: 2512-2519.
80. Bangalore DV, McGlynn W, Scott DD. Effect of beta-cyclodextrin in improving the correlation between lycopene concentration and ORAC values. J Agric Food Chem 2005; 53(6): 1878-1883.
81. Lussignoli S, Fraccaroli M, Andrioli G, Brocco G, Bellavite PA. Microplate-based colorimetric assay of the total peroryl radical trapping capability of human plasma. Analytical Biochemistry1999; 269: 38-44.
82. Kampa M, Nistikaki A, Tsaousis V, Maliaraki N, Notas G, Castanas EA. New automated method for the determination of the total antioxidant capacity (TAC) of human plasma, bases on the crocin bleanching assay. BMC. Clinical Pathology 2002, 2.
83. Tubaro F, Micossi E, Ursini F. The antioxidant capacity of complex mixtures by kinetic analysis of crocin bleaching inhibition. J Am Oil Chem Soc 1996; 73. 173–179.
84. Benzie IFF, Strain JJ. The ferric reducing ability of plasma (FRAP) as a measure of “antioxidant Power”: The FRAP assay. Anal Biochem 1996, 239: 70.
85. Takeoka GR, Dao L, Flessa S, Gillespie DM, Jewell WT, Huebner B, Bertow D, Ebeler SE. Processing effects on lycopene content and antioxidant activity of tomatoes. J Agric Food Chem 2001; 49: 3713-3717.

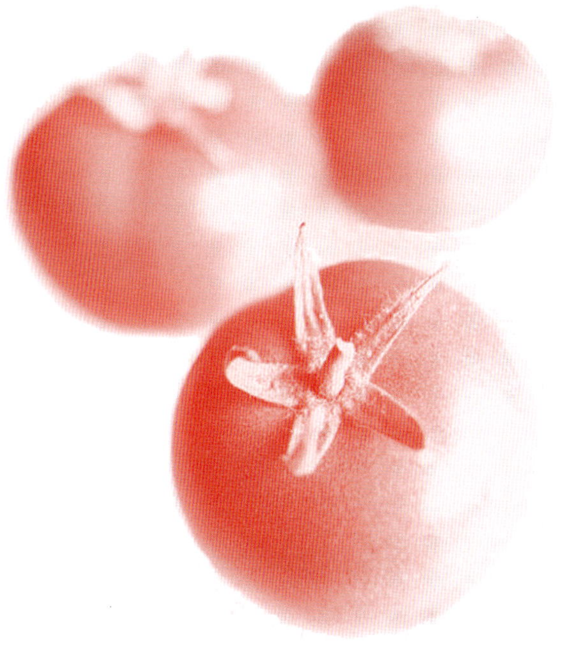

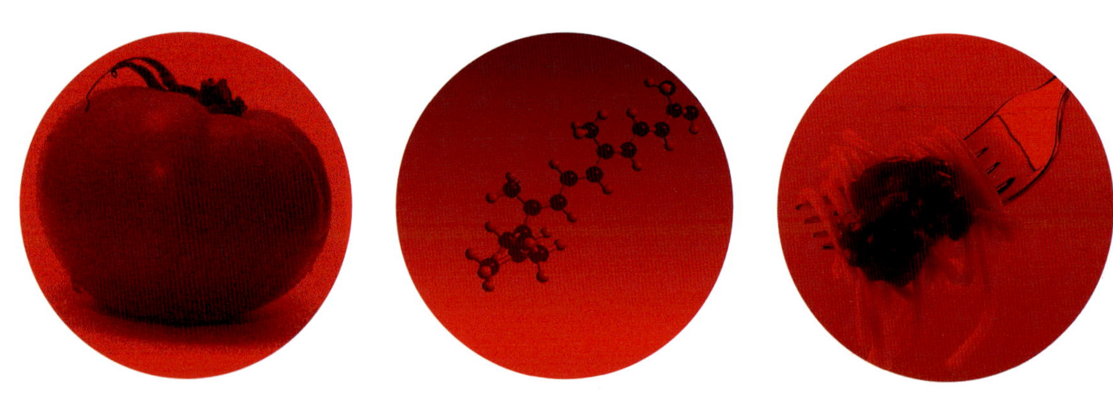

Mechanisms of Action of Lycopene

Dr. David Heber
Professor of Medicine and Director,
UCLA Center for Human Nutrition
David Geffen School of Medicine
University of California, Los Angeles
United States of America

Abstract

Tomatoes are the fourth most commonly eaten fresh vegetable and the most commonly eaten canned vegetable in the United States. Dietary intakes of tomatoes and tomato products containing lycopene have been shown to be associated with decreased risks of chronic diseases including cancer and cardiovascular diseases in numerous studies. Lycopene functions as a very potent antioxidant, and this is clearly a major mechanism of lycopene action. However, evidence is accumulating for other mechanisms as well. Lycopene at physiological concentrations can inhibit human cancer cell growth by interfering with growth factor receptor signaling and cell cycle progression specifically in prostate cancer cells without evidence of toxic effects or apoptosis of cells. Studies using human and animal cells have identified a gene, connexin 43, whose expression is upregulated by lycopene and which allows direct intercellular gap junctional communication (GJC). GJC is deficient in many human tumors and its restoration or upregulation is associated with decreased proliferation. The combination of low concentrations of lycopene with 1,25-dihydroxyvitamin D3 exhibits a synergistic effect on cell proliferation and differentiation and an additive effect on cell cycle progression in the HL-60 promyelocytic leukemia cell line, suggesting some interaction at a nuclear or subcellular level.

The combination of lycopene and lutein synergistically interact as antioxidants, and this may relate to specific positioning of different carotenoids in membranes. There is a growing body of evidence that carotenoids have unexpected biologic effects in experimental systems, some of which may contribute to their cancer preventive properties in models of carcinogenesis.

Consideration of solubility *in vitro*, comparison with doses achieved in humans by dietary means, interactions with other phytochemicals, and other potential mechanisms such as stimulation of xenobiotic metabolism, inhibition of cholesterogenesis, modulation of cyclooxygenase pathways, and inhibition of inflammation may also be important.

INTRODUCTION

Phytochemicals from fruits, vegetables, and whole grains play an important role in human health. Among the thousands of naturally occurring phytochemicals, tomato lycopene is a red pigment which can also be synthesized by other red plants and red microorganisms but not by animals. Lycopene is a carotenoid which has the structure of an acyclic isomer of ß-carotene and is found in combination with phytoene and phytofluene on the chromoplast of tomatoes where it has a role in protecting the plant against heat-mediated oxidant damage.

Once digested or heat-processed, the lycopene and related carotenoids become biologically available. Since lycopene lacks the ß-ionone ring structure of ß-carotene, it cannot form vitamin A (1). The cellular and molecular mechanisms of action of tomato lycopene can be classified into the categories of antioxidant activities or mechanisms beyond antioxidation.

ANTIOXIDANT MECHANISMS

Antioxidant mechanisms include the inactivation of reactive oxygen species which can significantly delay or prevent oxidative damage. Antioxidants such as vitamin E, vitamin C, polyphenols and carotenoids are available from food. Antioxidants also interact with the antioxidant response elements in the nucleus to activate antioxidant defense mechanisms based on the expression of enzymes including superoxide dismutase, catalase and glutathione peroxidase within cells. The body has numerous antioxidant defense mechanisms with a high degree of redundancy. However, under certain conditions it is possible to demonstrate the dependence of biological systems on the intake of antioxidants including carotenoids such as lycopene.

Lycopene is one of the most potent antioxidants (2-5), with a singlet-oxygen-quenching ability twice as high as that of ß-carotene and 10 times higher than that of α-tocopherol (5). Lycopene and other carotenoids are found to concentrate in low-density and very-low-density lipoprotein fractions of the serum (6). Lycopene can trap singlet oxygen and reduce mutagenesis in the Ames test. The antioxidant activity of carotenoids in multilamellar liposomes has been assayed by inhibition of formation of thiobarbituric acid-reactive substances (7). In this assay, lycopene has been demonstrated to be the most potent antioxidant with the ranking: lycopene > α-tocopherol > α-carotene > ß-cryptoxanthin > zeaxanthin > ß-carotene > lutein.

Mixtures of carotenoids were more effective than the single compounds. This synergistic effect was most pronounced when lycopene or lutein was present. The superior protection of mixtures may be related to specific positioning of different carotenoids in membranes.

The antioxidant properties of tomato products providing dietary lycopene including tomato juice, spaghetti sauce, and tomato oleoresin were studied in 19 healthy human volunteers using a randomized, crossover design in which each source of lycopene was administered for 1 week (8). Blood samples were collected at the end of each treatment. Serum lycopene was extracted and measured by high-performance liquid chromatography (HPLC) using an absorbance detector. Serum thiobarbituric acid-reactive substances, protein thiols, and 8-oxodeoxyguanosine contents of lymphocyte DNA were assayed to measure lipid, protein, and DNA oxidation.

Lycopene was the major carotenoid present in the serum. Dietary supplementation of lycopene resulted in a significant increase in serum lycopene level and diminished amounts of serum thiobarbituric acid-reactive substances. Although not statistically significant, a tendency of lowered protein and DNA oxidation was observed. There was also indication that the lycopene levels increased in a dose-dependent manner in the case of spaghetti sauce and tomato oleoresin. These results indicate that lycopene absorbed from tomato products may act as an *in vivo* antioxidant.

Lycopene may prevent carcinogenesis and atherogenesis by protecting critical cellular biomolecules, including lipids, lipoproteins, proteins and DNA (9-11). In healthy human subjects, lycopene- or tomato-free diets resulted in loss of lycopene and increased lipid oxidation (12) whereas dietary supplementation with lycopene for 1 week increased serum lycopene levels and reduced endogenous levels of oxidation of lipids, proteins, lipoproteins and DNA (9,10).

Tissue-specific lycopene distribution may be important in its mechanisms of action as an antioxidant. Lycopene is found to concentrate in the adrenal gland, testes, liver and prostate gland, where it is the most prominent carotenoid (13-16). Patients with prostate cancer were found to have low levels of lycopene and high levels of oxidation of serum lipids and proteins (17).

MECHANISMS OF ACTION IN CANCER BEYOND ANTIOXIDATION

There are several mechanisms by which tomato lycopene may inhibit tumorigenesis. Lycopene has been found to inhibit proliferation of several types of cancer cells, including those of breast, lung, and endometrium. Studies using human and animal cells have identified a gene, connexin 43, whose expression is upregulated by lycopene and which allows direct intercellular gap junctional communication (GJC). GJC is deficient in many human tumors and its restoration or upregulation is associated with decreased proliferation (18,19). This effect appears unrelated to antioxidant properties, since antioxidants without carotenoid properties such as methyl-bixin and alpha-tocopherol do not increase the expression of this gene.

The action is not believed to be via effects mediated by retinoid receptors, since the active carotenoid canthaxanthin does not induce the vitamin A-inducible gene retinoic acid receptor-beta but induces connexin 43 as does lycopene. Connexin 43 is the first carotenoid-inducible gene described in mammals.

In vitro studies demonstrate that lycopene reduces cellular proliferation in various cancer cell lines induced by insulin-like growth factors (20). Lycopene is hypothesized to suppress carcinogen-induced phosphorylation of regulatory proteins such as p53 and Rb antioncogenes and stop cell division at the G_0-G_1 cell cycle phase (20). The growth stimulation of MCF-7 mammary cancer cells by insulin-like growth factor 1(IGF-I) was markedly reduced by physiological concentrations of lycopene. The inhibitory effects of lycopene on MCF-7 cell growth were not accompanied by apoptotic or necrotic cell death, as determined by annexin V binding to plasma membrane and propidium iodide staining of nuclei in unfixed cells.

Lycopene treatment markedly reduced the IGF-I stimulation of tyrosine phosphorylation of insulin receptor substrate 1 and the binding capacity of the AP-1 transcription complex. These effects were not associated with changes in the number or affinity of IGF-I receptors, but with an increase in membrane-associated IGF-binding proteins, which were previously shown in different cancer cells to negatively regulate IGF-I receptor activation. The inhibitory effect of lycopene on IGF signaling was associated with suppression of IGF-stimulated cell cycle progression of serum-starved, synchronized cells. Moreover, in cells synchronized by mimosine treatment, lycopene delayed cell cycle progression after release from the mimosine block.

Collectively, the above data suggest that the inhibitory effects of lycopene on MCF-7 cell growth were not due to the toxicity of the carotenoid, but to interference in

IGF-I receptor signaling and cell cycle progression. The significance of this finding for cancer prevention is related to independent epidemiological findings that elevated IGF-I levels increase lifetime risks of breast and prostate cancer. IGF-I is manufactured in the liver as the result of growth hormone stimulation, but circulating levels of IGF-I are modulated by nutritional status. Undernutrition is associated with reduced levels, whereas obesity in childhood is associated with markedly increased circulating levels of IGF-I.

If lycopene interference with IGF-I stimulation of tumor cell growth is confirmed in clinical studies, this would provide a strong rationale for recommending increased intake of tomato products for cancer prevention.

The HL-60 promyelocytic leukemia cell line has been extensively studied with a variety of differentiating and antiproliferative agents. In studies (21) by Amir *et al.*, lycopene resulted in a concentration-dependent reduction in HL-60 cell growth as measured by [^{3}H]thymidine incorporation and cell counting.

This effect was accompanied by inhibition of cell cycle progression in the G_0/G_1 phase as measured by flow cytometry. Lycopene alone induced cell differentiation as measured by phorbol ester-dependent reduction of nitroblue tetrazolium and expression of the cell surface antigen CD14. The combination of low concentrations of lycopene with 1,25-dihydroxyvitamin D3 exhibited a synergistic effect on cell proliferation and differentiation and an additive effect on cell cycle progression (22).

Such synergistic antiproliferative and differentiating effects of lycopene and other compounds found in the diet and in plasma suggest that phytochemicals such as vitamin D and lycopene, with separate modes of action, may unexpectedly combine to promote anticancer effects not seen with either agent alone. Because high doses of 1,25-dihydroxyvitamin D3 are required for antiproliferative effects and these doses are complicated by serious hypercalcemia, one solution may be to combine multiple compounds, including lycopene, in prevention efforts.

Astorg and colleagues (23) demonstrated that lycopene can modulate the liver metabolizing enzyme, cytochrome P450 2E1. This xenobiotic metabolizing action may be an underlying mechanism of protection against carcinogen-induced preneoplastic lesions..

Tomato lycopene may also be beneficial to immune surveillance of tumor cells. Regulation of intrathymic T-cell differentiation was suggested to be the mechanism for suppression of mammary tumour growth by lycopene treatments in SHN retired mice (24,25).

MODULATION OF CHOLESTEROL METABOLISM

Lycopene accumulates during tomato ripening as the result of down-regulation of the gene lycopene epsilon-cyclase which converts lycopene to ß-carotene. Both ß-carotene and lycopene share similar initial synthetic pathways with cholesterol, which is synthesized in animal but not in plant cells. Some of the intermediary metabolites in these pathways called isoprenoids are found in large quantities in numerous fruits and can exert negative feedback on cholesterogenesis independent of direct inhibition of HMG-CoA reductase. The observations of Elson, Mo and co-workers (27) have implications for both heart disease risk reduction and inhibition of carcinogenesis.

Cancer cells have abnormal cholesterol biosynthetic pathways that are resistant to down-regulation by cholesterol, and farnesylation is a key process in oncogene activation. Supplementation with multiple carotenoids from fruits and vegetables, including tomato products, may help to prevent common forms of cancer via this pathway as well as the others reviewed above.

Lycopene also has been shown to act as a hypocholesterolemic agent by inhibiting HMG-CoA (3-hydroxy-3-methylglutaryl- coenzyme A) reductase. Fuhrman *et al*.(28) examined the effect of carotenoids on macrophage cholesterol metabolism in comparison with the effect of low-density lipoprotein (LDL) cholesterol and of the cholesterol synthesis inhibitor, fluvastatin. In J-774 A. 1 macrophage cell line, *de novo* cellular cholesterol synthesis from [^{3}H]acetate, but not from [^{14}C] mevalonate, was suppressed by 63% and by 73% following cell incubation with ß-carotene or lycopene (10 μ*M*), respectively, in comparison with a 90% and 91% inhibition by LDL (100 μg of cholesterol) or by fluvastatin (10 μg/ml), respectively. However, unlike LDL-derived cholesterol, which also suppresses macrophage LDL receptor activity, lycopene and ß-carotene augmented the activity of the macrophage LDL receptor, similar to the effect of fluvastatin.

In agreement with these *in vitro* observations, dietary supplementation of lycopene (60 mg/day) to six men for a 3-month period resulted in a significant 14% reduction in their plasma LDL cholesterol concentrations. These findings suggest that dietary supplementation of carotenoids may act as moderate hypocholesterolemic agents, secondary to their inhibitory effect on macrophage 3-hydroxy-3-methyl glutaryl coenzyme A (HMGCoA) reductase, the rate-limiting enzyme in cholesterol synthesis.

ANTI-INFLAMMATORY ACTIONS OF LYCOPENE

In a cross-sectional study (29), the acute phase response of inflammation, as defined by an elevation of C-reactive protein, was associated with suppressed circulating levels of antioxidants in a population of 85 Catholic sisters (nuns) 77–99 years of age. The presence of an acute phase response was associated with an expected significant decrease in the serum concentrations of albumin ($P < 0.001$) and thyroxine-binding prealbumin ($P < 0.001$), as well as an expected significant increase in copper ($P < 0.001$) and fibrinogen ($P = 0.003$). In addition, there was a significant decrease in the plasma concentrations of lycopene ($P = 0.03$), α-carotene ($P = 0.02$), ß-carotene ($P = 0.02$), and total carotenoids ($P = 0.01$). This decrease in circulating antioxidants may further compromise antioxidant status and may increase oxidative stress and damage in the elderly with inflammatory conditions.In nine adult women (30), the consumption of 25 g of tomato puree (containing 7 mg of lycopene and 0.3 mg of ß-carotene) for 14 consecutive days increased plasma and lymphocyte carotenoid concentration, and this was related to an improvement in lymphocyte resistance to an oxidative stress (500 µ*M*/l hydrogen peroxide for 5 min).

Before and after the period of tomato intake, carotenoid concentrations were analyzed by HPLC and lymphocyte resistance to oxidative stress by the Comet assay, which detects DNA strand breaks. Intake of tomato puree increased plasma ($P < 0.001$) and lymphocyte ($P < 0.005$) lycopene concentration and reduced lymphocyte DNA damage by approximately 50% ($P < 0.0001$). ß-Carotene concentration increased in plasma ($P < 0.05$) but not in lymphocytes after tomato puree consumption. An inverse relationship was found between plasma lycopene concentration ($r = -0.82$, $P < 0.0001$) and lymphocyte lycopene concentration ($r = -0.62$, $P < 0.01$) and the oxidative DNA damage. These data suggest that small amounts of tomato puree or other processed tomato products such as juices, soups, or pasta sauces added to the diet over a short period can increase carotenoid concentrations and the resistance of lymphocytes to oxidative stress.

In one recent study (31), the normal diets of human volunteers were supplemented with either 15 mg/day ß-carotene ($n = 25$), lycopene ($n = 23$), or lutein ($n = 21$) for 26 days in three independent double-blind, placebo-controlled supplementation studies. Supplementation with ß-carotene increased plasma linoleic acid, but left the polyunsaturated:saturated (P:S) fatty acid ratio unaltered. In contrast, supplementation with lycopene reduced linoleic acid, which resulted in a large decrease in the P:S ratio. Lutein supplementation had no effect. It was concluded that neither ß-carotene, lycopene, nor lutein supplementation engender antioxidant effects that lead to the widespread general conservation of plasma polyunsaturated fatty acids (PUFAs). ß-Carotene and lycopene supplementation appear to interact with the metabolism of linoleic acid, the "essential" fatty acid, resulting in either an increase (ß-carotene) or decrease (lycopene) in its plasma concentration. Alterations in plasma 18:2 or P:S ratios could ultimately lead to changes in tissue cellular membrane composition and hence to alterations in eicosanoid biosynthesis. More research is needed on the effects of lycopene and other carotenoids on xenobiotic metabolism (32) and on its effects on inducible cyclo-oxygenase activity.

CONCLUSIONS

The current dietary recommendation to increase the consumption of fruits and vegetables rich in antioxidants has generated interest in the role of lycopene in disease prevention. However, the evidence thus far is mainly suggestive, and the underlying mechanisms are not clearly understood. Further research is critical to elucidate the role of lycopene and to formulate guidelines for healthy eating and disease prevention. Areas for further study include epidemiological investigations based on serum lycopene levels, bioavailability and effects of dietary factors, long-term dietary intervention studies, metabolism and isomerization of lycopene and their biological significance, interaction with other carotenoids and antioxidants, and mechanism of disease prevention. Of particular importance, is an improved understanding of the mechanisms of action of lycopene in cancer chemoprevention and in nutritional strategies for cancer prevention.

There is clear evidence from epidemiologic studies that the intake of 400–600 g per day of fruits and vegetables is associated with a reduced risk of common aerodigestive cancers (33). Recent epidemiological studies indicate that increased serum α-carotene and lycopene levels are associated with a reduced risk of lung cancer, even among smokers (34). This observation is consistent with the lack of effect of smoking on serum lycopene levels while markedly decreasing ß-carotene levels. This suggests a special protective role in lung cancer just as the localization of lycopene to the prostate gland suggests a special protective role there. Fruit and vegetable interventions at the level of 500 g per day are practical and result in significant changes in the levels of biochemical markers such as folic acid and homocysteine (35). The emerging science suggests that it is now time to make dietary changes as the scientific evidence continues to build (36).

REFERENCES :

1. Stahl W, Sies H. Lycopene: A biologically important carotenoid for humans? Arch *Biochem Biophys* 1996;336:1-9.
2. Miller NJ, Sampson J, Candeias LP, Bramley PM, Rice-Evans CA. Antioxidant activities of carotenes and xanthophylls. FEBS Lett 1996;384:240-6.
3. Mortensen A, Skibsted LH. Relative stability of carotenoid radical cations and homologue tocopheroxyl radicals. A real time kinetic study of antioxidant hierarchy. *FEBS Lett* 997;417:261-6.
4. Woodall AA, Lee SWM, Weesie RJ, Jackson MJ, Britton G. Oxidation of carotenoids by free radicals: relationship between structure and reactivity. *Biochim Biophys Acta* 1997;1336:33-42.
5. DiMascio P, Kaiser S, Sies H. Lycopene as the most effective biological carotenoid singlet oxygen quencher. *Arch Biochem Biophys* 1989;274:532-8.
6. Clinton SK. Lycopene: chemistry, biology, and implications for human health and disease. *Nutr Rev* 1998;56:35-51.
7. Stahl W, Junghans A, de Boer B, Driomina ES, Briviba K, Sies H. Carotenoid mixtures protect multilamellar liposomes against oxidative damage: synergistic effects of lycopene and lutein. FEBS Lett 427: 305—308, 1998.
8. Rao AV, Agarwal S. Bioavailability and in vivo antioxidant properties of lycopene from tomato products and their possible role in the prevention of cancer. Nutr Cancer 31:199—203, 1998.
9. Agarwal S, Rao AV. Tomato lycopene and low density lipoprotein oxidation: a human dietary intervention study. *Lipids* 1998;33:981-4.
10. Rao AV, Agarwal S. Bioavailability and in vivo antioxidant properties of lycopene from tomato products and their possible role in the prevention of cancer. *Nutr Cancer* 1998;31:199-203.
11. Pool-Zobel BL, Bub A, Muller H, Wollowski I, Rechkemmer G. Consumption of vegetables reduces genetic damage in humans: first results of a human intervention trial with carotenoid-rich foods. *Carcinogenesis* 1997;18:1847-50.
12. Rao AV, Agarwal S. Effect of diet and smoking on serum lycopene and lipid peroxidation. *Nutr Res* 1998;18:713-21.
13. Stahl W, Schwarz W, Sundquist AR, Sies H. cis-trans Isomers of lycopene and betacarotene in human serum and tissues. *Arch Biochem Biophys* 1992;294:173-7.
14. Kaplan LA, Lau JM, Stein EA. Carotenoid composition, concentrations and relationships in various human organs. *Clin Physiol Biochem* 1990;8:1-10.
15. Schmitz HH, Poor CL, Wellman RB, Erdman JW Jr. Concentrations of selected carotenoids and vitamin A in human liver, kidney and lung tissue. J Nutr 1991;121:1613-21.
16. Nierenberg DW, Nann SL. A method for determining concentrations of retinol,tocopherol, and five carotenoids in human plasma and tissue samples. *Am J Clin Nutr* 1992;56:417-26.
17. Rao AV, Fleshner N, Agarwal S. Serum and tissue lycopene and biomarkers of oxidation in prostate cancer patients: a case control study. Nutr Cancer 1999;33: 159-64.
18. Zhang LX, Cooney RV, Bertram JS. Carotenoids enhance gap junctional communication and inhibit lipid peroxidation in C3H/10T1/2 cells: relationship to their cancer chemopreventive action. *Carcinogenesis* 1991;12:2109-14.

19. Zhang LX, Cooney RV, Bertram JS. Carotenoids up-regulate connexin43 gene expression independent of their provitamin A or antioxidant properties. *Cancer Res* 1992;52:5707-12.
20. Levy J, Bosin E, Feldmen B, Giat Y, Miinster A, Danilenko M, et al. Lycopene is a more potent inhibitor of human cancer cell proliferation than either α-carotene or β-carotene. *Nutr Cancer* 1995;24:257-66.
21. Amir H, Karas M, Giat J, Danilenko M, Levy R, Yermiahu T, Levy J, Sharoni Y. Lycopene and 1,25-dihydroxyvitamin D3 cooperate in the inhibition of cell cycle progression and induction of differentiation in HL-60 leukemic cells. Nutr Cancer 33:105–112, 1999.
22. Karas M, Amir H, Fishman D, Danilenko M, Segal S, Nahum A, Koifmann A, Giat Y, Levy J, Sharoni Y. Lycopene interferes with cell cycle progression and insulin-like growth factor I signaling in mammary cancer cells. Nutr Cancer 36:101–111, 2000.
23. Astorg P, Gradelet S, Berges R, Suschetet M. Dietary lycopene decreases the initiation of liver preneoplastic foci by diethylnitrosamine in the rat. *Nutr Cancer* 1997;29(1):60-8.
24. Nagasawa H, Mitamura T, Sakamoto S, Yamamoto K. Effects of lycopene on spontaneous mammary tumour development in SHN virgin mice. *Anticancer Res* 1995;15:1173-8.
25. Kobayashi T, Iijima K, Mitamura T, Toriizuka K, Cyong JC, Nagasawa H. Effects of lycopene, a carotenoid, on intrathymic T cell differentiation and peripheral CD4/CD8 ratio in a high mammary tumor strain of SHN retired mice. *Anticancer Drugs* 1996;7:195-8.
26. Ronen G, Cohen M, Zamir D, Hirschberg J. Regulation of carotenoid biosynthesis during tomato fruit development: expression of the gene for lycopene epsilon-cyclase is down-regulated during ripening and is elevated in the mutant . Plant J 17:341–351, 1999.
27. Elson CE, Peffley DM, Hentosh P, Mo H. Isoprenoid-mediated inhibition of mevalonate synthesis: potential application to cancer. Proc Soc Exp Biol Med 22:294–310, 1999.
28. Fuhramn B, Elis A, Aviram M. Hypocholesterolemic effect of lycopene and β-carotene is related to suppression of cholesterol synthesis and augmentation of LDL receptor activity in macrophage. *Biochem Biophys Res Commun* 1997;233: 658-62.
29. Boosalis MG, Snowdon DA, Tully CL, Gross MD. Acute phase response and plasma carotenoid concentrations in older women: findings from the nun study. Nutrition 12:475–478, 1996.
30. Porrini M, Riso P. Lymphocyte lycopene concentration and DNA protection from oxidative damage is increased in women after a short period of tomato consumption. J Nutr 130:189–192, 2000.
31. Wright AJ, Hughes DA, Bailey AL, Southon S. β-Carotene and lycopene, but not lutein, supplementation changes the plasma fatty acid profile of healthy male non-smokers. J Lab Clin Med 134:592–598, 1999.
32. Heber D, Go VLW. Gene-nutrient interaction and the xenobiotic hypothesis of cancer. In: Heber D, Blackburn GL, Go VLW, Eds. Nutritional Oncology. San Diego, CA: Academic Press, 1999.
33. World Cancer Research Fund: American Institute for Cancer Research. Food, nutrition, and the prevention of cancer: A global perspective. Washington, DC: American Institute for Cancer Research, 1997.
34. Heber D. Colorful cancer prevention: α-carotene, lycopene, and lung cancer. Am J Clin Nutr 72:901–902, 2000.

35. Broekmans WM, Klopping-Ketelaars IA, Schuurman CR, Verhagen H, van den Berg H, Kok FJ, von Poppel G. Fruits and vegetables increase plasma carotenoids and vitamins and decrease homocysteine in humans. J Nutr 130:1578—1583, 2000.
36. Heber D, Bowerman S. What Color is Your Diet? New York: Harper-Collins/Regan Books, 2001.

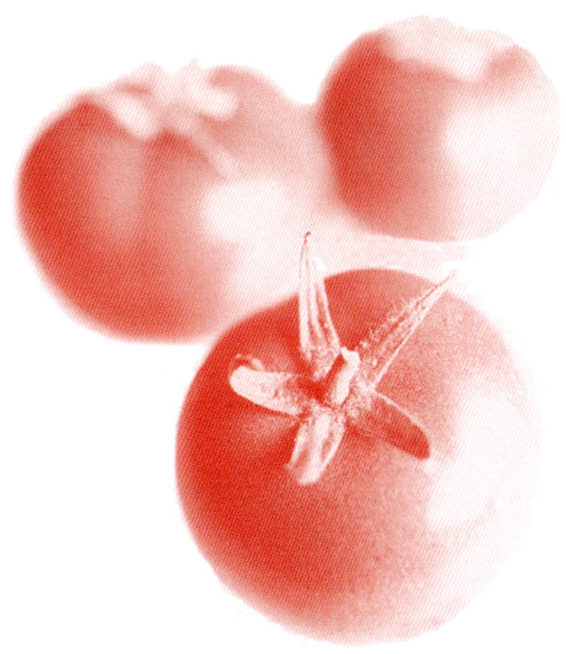

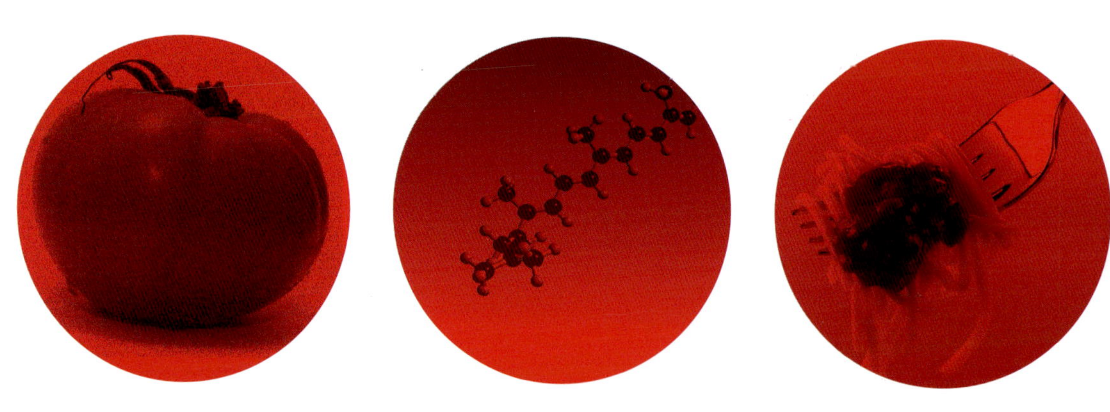

Why Lycopene is Beneficial Against Chronic Disease:

The Molecular Mechanisms

Dr. R. Edge
Dr. T.G. Truscott
School of Physical and Geographical Sciences,
Keele University
Free Radical Research Facility,
CCLRC, Daresbury Laboratory,
Warrington, United Kingdom

Abstract

Lycopene, like all other dietary carotenoids, reacts with free radicals via at least three different processes: electron transfer, hydrogen atom transfer and addition. In all cases the resulting product/s are themselves free radicals (i.e. contain an odd electron) and may well be reactive (i.e. oxidising). This is particularly important following electron transfer because the product, a carotenoid radical cation, is known to be a strongly oxidising species. This review describes several reactions of such carotene (lycopene) radical cations e.g. with amino acids and vitamin C. Another important reaction of carotenoids, including lycopene, is the extremely efficient quenching of the potentially damaging 'singlet oxygen'. In environments which model *in vivo* membranes both lycopene and ß-carotene are efficient singlet oxygen quenchers but there is no difference between the efficiency of these carotenoids in contrast to some earlier claims that lycopene is the most efficient singlet oxygen quencher.

I. INTRODUCTION

Recent evidence suggests that lycopene, the red colourant in tomatoes, gives protection against many chronic diseases including prostate cancer, heart disease and possibly age-related blindness (1-4). However, the understanding of how this protection arises (on a molecular basis) is far from complete.

Furthermore, while lycopene may accumulate to some extent in some organs, such as the prostate, it also offers protection against age-related macular degeneration (AMD), the major cause of blindness in old age in the developed world, even though lycopene does not accumulate in the eye. Mechanisms, which may explain the benefits of lycopene in protection against these and other (5) chronic diseases, are the topic of this paper.

Lycopene is one member of a group of naturally occurring highly coloured pigments called carotenoids. Carotenoids are present in many fruits and vegetables and there are well over 600 carotenoids but only about 40 of these are consumed as dietary carotenoids.

Important naturally occurring dietary carotenoids include astaxanthin (responsible for the pink colour of salmon), canthaxanthin and ß-carotene (both often used as food colourants) and lutein and zeaxanthin which accumulate in our eyes and are thought to protect the eyes from the harmful effects of blue light. The depletion of lutein and zeaxanthin may well be related to the onset of AMD. Many of these carotenoids are widely distributed throughout fruits and vegetables. On the other hand lycopene is not widely distributed and well over 90% of lycopene consumption comes from the tomato. Interestingly, the best dietary source is cooked tomatoes rather than fresh tomatoes, the cooking process aiding the bio-availability of the lycopene from the fruits (6).

Lycopene has been studied for about 100 years with the chemical structure being established about 70 years ago. This structure, together with that of several other important carotenoids is given in Figure 1.

The chemical structure of lycopene is quite different from other such carotenoids. All other dietary carotenoids have structures that include terminal rings (of six carbon atoms) but lycopene contains no such rings. It is also noteworthy that the carotenoids that accumulate in the eye, zeaxanthin and lutein, have –OH groups on these terminal rings. This structural feature may be important to their role in protecting the eye from damage by oxy-radicals. Subsequent early work established the isomerisation processes (change of shape) and other parameters such as stability and more recently the human tissue concentrations of lycopene. For a review of such information see Nguyan and Schwartz (7).

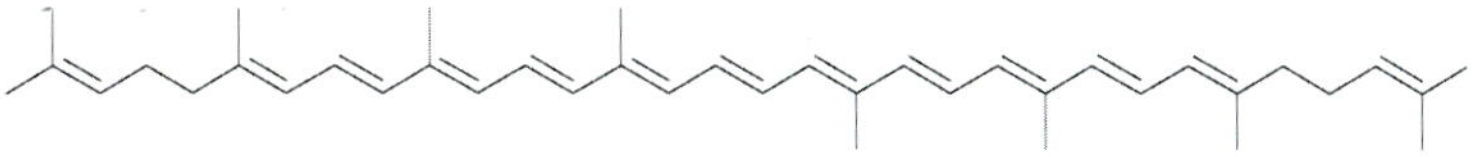

Lycopene

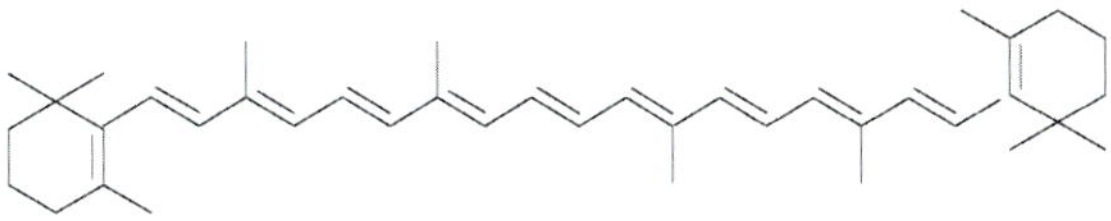

β-Carotene

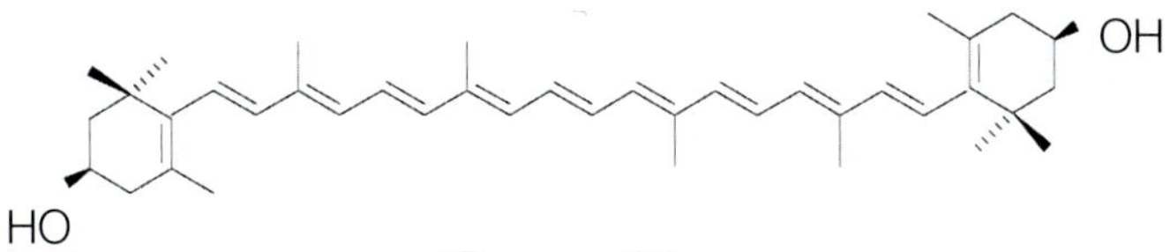

OH
HO
Zeaxanthin

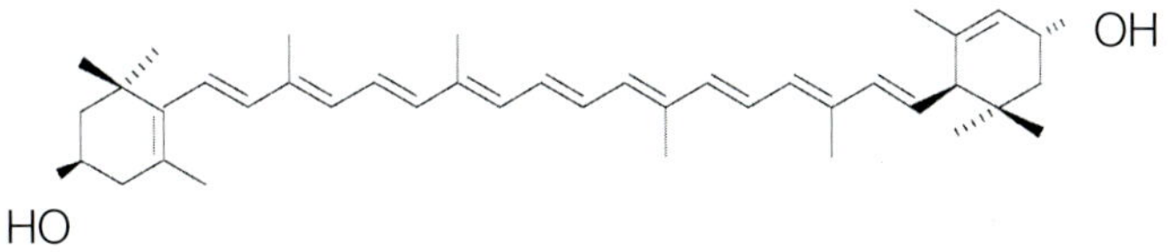

OH
HO
Lutein

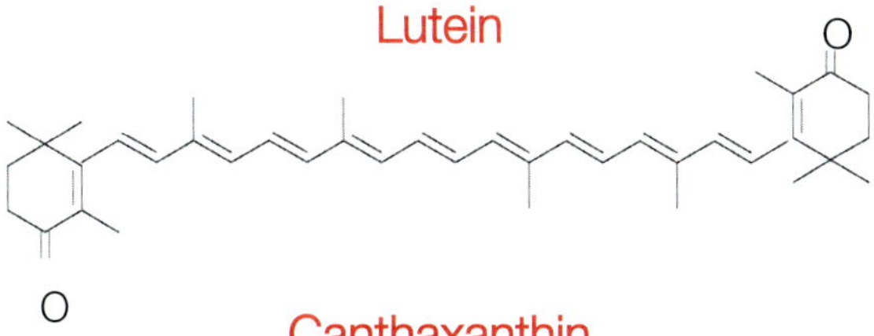

O
O
Canthaxanthin

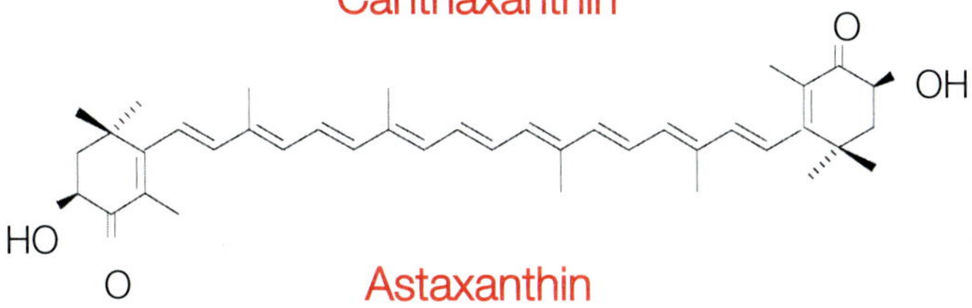

O
OH
HO
O
Astaxanthin

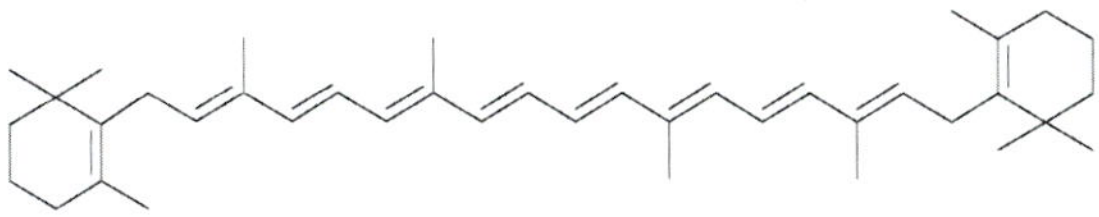

7,7 -Dihydro-β-carotene

Fig 1: Chemical Structures of Dietary Cartenoids

II. MOLECULAR MECHANISMS INVOLVING FREE RADICALS

We have already noted that there is much evidence for a beneficial value of dietary lycopene in preventing prostate cancer, heart disease and AMD. Furthermore, Gerster (5) has reviewed the beneficial role of lycopene in protection against a wider range of chronic diseases. The question we now address is how does this protection arise, that is, what are the molecular mechanisms underlying the protection against many chronic diseases afforded by dietary lycopene?

Two quite different mechanisms have been suggested to account for the beneficial value of carotenoids in general, (i) the anti-oxidant reactions involving removal of damaging free radicals and the quenching of 'singlet oxygen' and (ii) gap junction potentials (8). However, (ii) does not account for the advantage of lycopene over all other dietary carotenoids and will not be considered further.

We start with some simple definitions of free radicals and anti- and pro-oxidants: A free radical is a species with an 'odd' (usually called an unpaired) electron. A free radical is usually very reactive (damaging) because it tries to either lose an electron or acquire an electron from another species, so that all electrons are paired.

An oxy-radical simply has the odd electron (usually shown as a dot) localised near an oxygen atom, e.g. alkylperoxyl radical may be written as $^{\bullet}O_2CH_2R$ and nitrogen dioxide as $NO_2^{\bullet}$.

There are several ways of defining anti- and pro-oxidants. It is simplest to note that an anti-oxidant reacts with a damaging oxy-radical to remove it from the body and hence protect the body from the initiation of disease, while a pro-oxidant reacts to increase damage – there has been much debate about the possible ability of ß-carotene to become a pro-oxidant under certain conditions see, for example (9). We also need to consider if the same could be true for lycopene.

At least three types of reaction between oxy-radicals and carotenoids (Car), such as lycopene, have been discussed.

Electron transfer	$R^{\bullet}$ + Car	→	R^{-} + $Car^{\bullet +}$
Hydrogen atom transfer	$R^{\bullet}$ + Car(H)	→	RH + $Car^{\bullet}$
Addition reactions	$R^{\bullet}$ + Car	→	$[R\cdots Car]^{\bullet}$

Furthermore, more than one type of addition product is possible.

II.A. Electron Transfer

One of the most important radical reactions is electron transfer between strongly oxidising radicals such as $NO_2^\bullet$ (which arise from environmental pollution and cigarette smoke) and lycopene. This type of reaction involves the oxy-radical taking an electron from lycopene and thus converting the oxy-radical to a harmless (non-radical) species as illustrated in the following equation (where L is lycopene):

Electron transfer $ROO^\bullet + L \rightarrow ROO^- + L^{\bullet+}$

It is important to note that the lycopene now contains an odd electron i.e. a lycopene radical has been generated (actually a lycopene radical with a positive charge which is called a lycopene radical cation).

The removal of the potentially damaging oxy-radical ($ROO^\bullet$) is clearly beneficial but we must consider what are the consequences of the production of $L^{\bullet+}$. This depends on the properties of $L^{\bullet+}$.

II.A.1. Properties of $L^{\bullet+}$ (and $Car^{\bullet+}$ in general)

The first property of interest is the lifetime of the carotenoid radical cations ($Car^{\bullet+}$ including $L^{\bullet+}$). If this is very short, it is very likely that such carotenoid radicals will not have time to undergo any reactions, that is, they would not be likely to cause any biological damage. However, we have been able to determine the lifetimes of several such carotenoid radical cations, including $L^{\bullet+}$ in liposomes and micelles which mimic cell membranes (measurements based on pulsed laser and pulsed electron beam (pulse radiolysis) methods, see (10) for details).

We reported a range of lifetimes ranging from about 1 millisecond to 1 second. While the reason for this range of lifetimes, rather than a single specific lifetime, is not entirely clear, there is ample time for $Car^{\bullet+}$ and $L^{\bullet+}$ to react with other molecules in the biological situation and hence they have the potential to cause biological damage.

II.A.2. Reactions of $L^{\bullet+}$ and $Car^{\bullet+}$

So far three reactions of potential biological/human importance have been established, each will be discussed in turn, these can be written as:

Reaction 1 $Car_1^{\bullet+} + Car_2 \rightarrow Car_1 + Car_2^{\bullet+}$

Reaction 2 $Car^{\bullet+}$ + amino acid (protein) → Car + oxidised amino acid (oxidised protein)

Reaction 3 $Car^{\bullet+}$ + ascorbic acid → Car + oxidised ascorbic acid

Reaction 1: $Car_1^{\bullet+} + Car_2 \rightarrow Car_1 + Car_2^{\bullet+}$

The efficiency of electron transfer reactions depend on the redox potentials involved. Pulse radiolysis (10) has allowed us to study pairs of carotenoids and observe the direction of the reaction e.g. to decide which of the following is the direction of electron transfer:

$L^{\bullet+} + Car \rightarrow L + Car^{\bullet+}$ or $Car^{\bullet+} + L \rightarrow Car + L^{\bullet+}$

Figure 2 shows a typical result in which the radical cation of lycopene abstracts an electron from astaxanthin and similar studies from many such pairs have allowed us to determine the direction of electron transfer for 6 important carotenoids, and suggested the order of relative reduction potentials as Astaxanthin > 8`-apo-ß-caroten-8`-al > canthaxanthin > lutein > zeaxanthin > ß-carotene > lycopene, as shown in Figure 3.

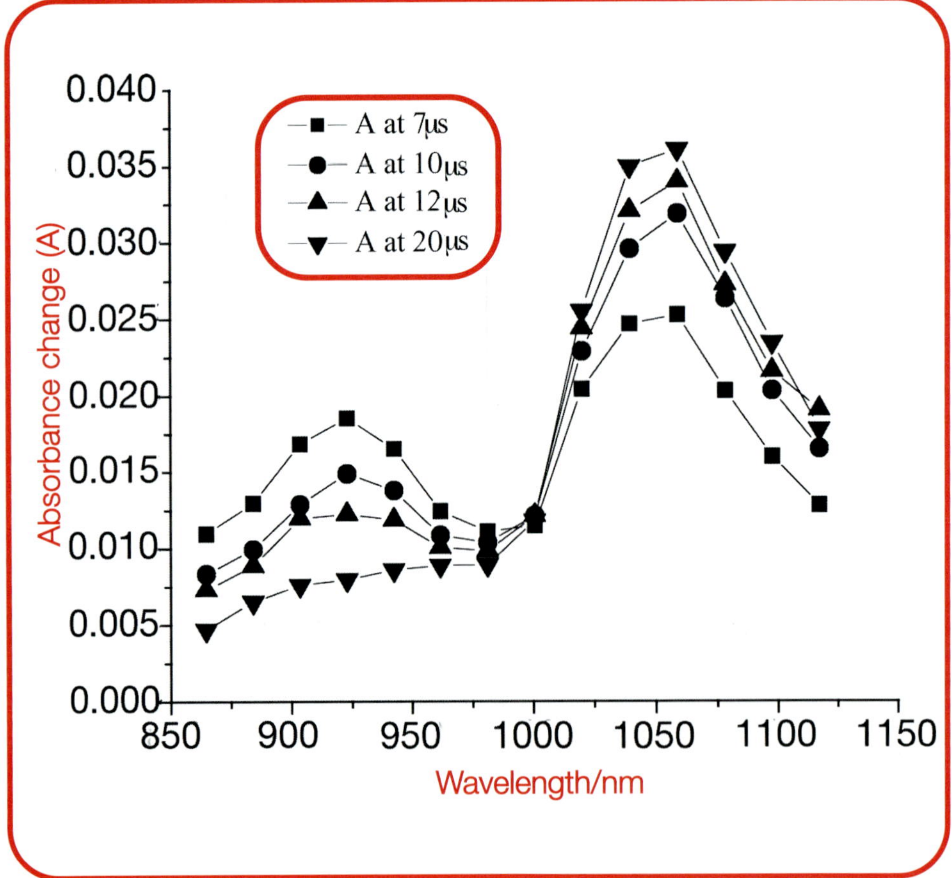

Fig 2: The decay of the astaxanthin radical cation at 925nm and the corresponding growth of the lycopene radical cation at 1050nm

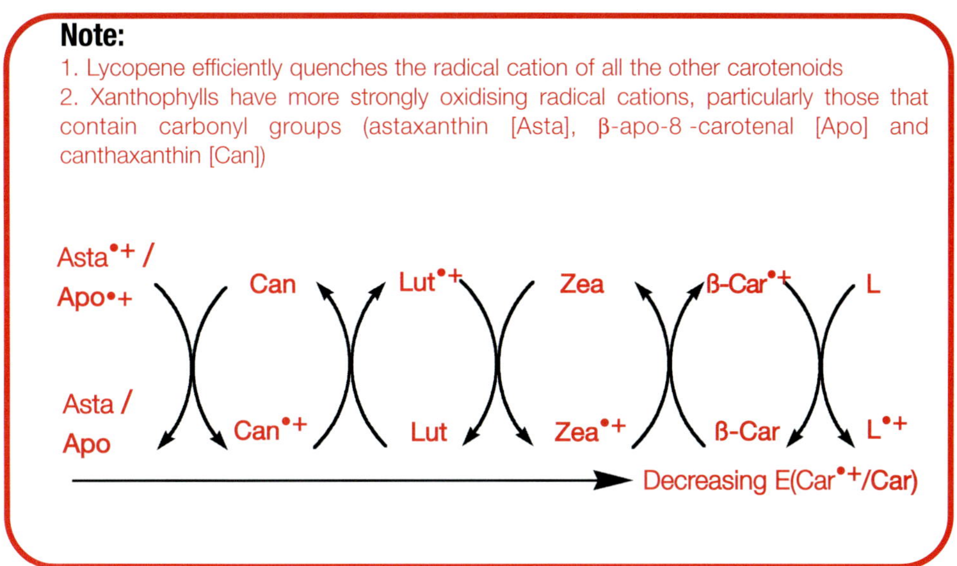

Fig 3: Order of 1-electron reduction potentials for some dietary carotenoids

As can be seen from the scheme (Figure 3) all other $Car^{\bullet +}$ are converted to Car by lycopene:

$$Car^{\bullet +} + L \rightarrow Car + L^{\bullet +}$$

that is, lycopene is the most easily oxidised of all the carotenoids. This suggests lycopene will be the most effective carotenoid at reacting with damaging oxy-radicals by electron transfer.

Such reactions of lycopene with the radical cations of the ocular carotenoids (zeaxanthin [Zea] and lutein [Lut]) allow us to speculate on a mechanism to explain the possible link between blindness in old age due to age-related macular degeneration (AMD) and low serum levels of lycopene. That is, to explain the protection due to lycopene even though it is well established that there is no lycopene in the macular (the so-called 'yellow spot') of the eye.

Zeaxanthin and lutein are taken in from the diet and, if they react with an oxy-radical, they may be converted to their respective radical cations:

$$ROO^{\bullet} + Lut \rightarrow ROO^{-} + Lut^{\bullet +} \text{ and } ROO^{\bullet} + Zea \rightarrow ROO^{-} + Zea^{\bullet +}$$

Neither $Lut^{\bullet+}$ nor $Zea^{\bullet+}$ are of value in protecting the eye, but they may be 'repaired' by lycopene (such repair is much less efficient with ß-carotene):

$Lut^{\bullet+} + L \rightarrow Lut + L^{\bullet+}$ and $Zea^{\bullet+} + L \rightarrow Zea + L^{\bullet+}$

Hence, lycopene may be able to repair 'spent' zeaxanthin and lutein so that they would again be of value in eye protection. (Possibly an alternative explanation is that trace amounts of other materials associated with lycopene supplementation are active in preventing AMD).

Reaction 2: $Car^{\bullet+}$ + amino acid → Car + oxidised amino acid

Such reactions may well lead to protein damage and hence are a route to disease initiation. The questions which arise are how reactive is $Car^{\bullet+}$ in general and, in particular, how reactive is $L^{\bullet+}$. Such reactivity is measured by obtaining the carotenoid redox potential.

By reacting the dietary carotenoids with molecules of known redox potential we have been able to obtain the corresponding value for six carotenoids and the value in each case is near +1 volt. This is rather high, and shows all $Car^{\bullet+}$ studied, including $L^{\bullet+}$, are strong oxidising agents. Lycopene has the lowest oxidising potential, as expected from the scheme in Figure 3. However, the range of values for all carotenoids, including lycopene, is 1020 ± 40mV.

Hence, all the dietary carotenoids, including lycopene, can be expected to oxidise several other biological targets. In fact, we have used our pulsed techniques (10) to directly demonstrate this with the amino acids tyrosine and cysteine, e.g:

$Car^{\bullet+}$ + tyrosine → Car + tyrosine oxidation products

and such reactions will lead to protein damage (e.g initiate cross-linking of tyrosine moieties in protein). This suggests that, unless there is a mechanism for removing $Car^{\bullet+}$, benefits of dietary carotenoids may be lost by reactions involving $Car^{\bullet+}$.

Reaction 3: $Car^{\bullet+}$ + vitamin C → Car + oxidised vitamin C

We have observed this reaction for all dietary carotenoids including lycopene. That is, vitamin C (ascorbic acid) is able to repair $Car^{\bullet+}$ (including $L^{\bullet+}$) and hence can prevent damage due to $Car^{\bullet+}$.

Lycopene (and all dietary carotenoids) are water insoluble and in the lipophilic environment of cell membranes. However, vitamin C/ascorbic acid is water-soluble and hence in the aqueous environment. Of course, the positive charge and radical nature of $L^{\bullet+}$ (or $Car^{\bullet+}$) will make it more polar than the 'parent' lycopene (or carotenoid) and this will allow $L^{\bullet+}$ to move/re-orientate so as to be nearer the cell membrane/water interface. Figure 4 illustrates this effect.

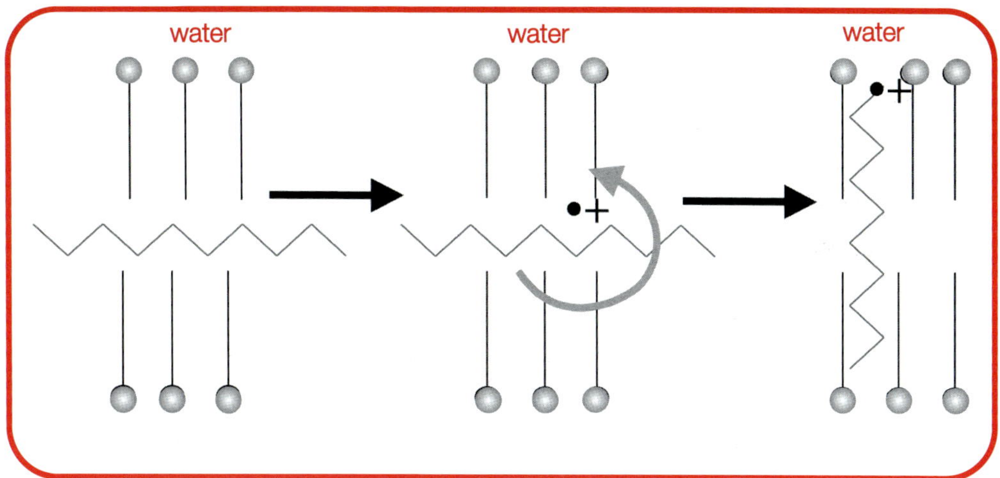

Fig 4: Suggested movement of $Car^{\bullet+}$ in lipid membranes

So, provided there is sufficient vitamin C present, the $L^{\bullet+}$ radical cation will be 'repaired' (i.e. converted back to the parent lycopene). This recycling of 'spent' lycopene clearly has two advantages: it removes the possibility of unwanted reactions of $L^{\bullet+}$ and improves the efficiency of the overall protection.

In an attempt to confirm such benefits of the combination of lycopene plus vitamin C, we have exposed human white blood cells to specific oxidising species which arise in cigarette smoke (e.g. $NO_2^{\bullet}$ and singlet oxygen) (11). Our volunteers (non-smokers, i.e. with adequate vitamin C) consumed 500 ml of pre-boiled tomato juice for 14 consecutive days before these experiments. We used a standard method to measure the cell membrane destruction (based on cell staining with eosin). Table 1 gives typical results and shows a high protection factor for human cells against $NO_2^{\bullet}$ by lycopene (or some component of the tomato juice) in the presence of adequate vitamin C. This protection was still present 4 days after the cessation of the consumption of the tomato juice.

Reactive Species	Tomato Juice	% Stained Cells	Protection Factor
$NO_2^{\bullet}$ $NO_2^{\bullet}$	No Yes	3.5 61.5	17.6
Singlet Oxygen Singlet Oxygen	No Yes	8.7 55.1	6.3

Table 1: Lymphocyte membrane destruction after exposure to $NO_2^{\bullet}$ or singlet oxygen, showing the protection factors afforded by the consumption of tomato juice

II.B. Other Radicals of Lycopene (and carotenoids in general)

Both neutral radicals ($L^•$) and addition radicals ($[R\cdots L]^•$) can arise (see II.A.1. above). These addition radicals are not well defined and ion-pairs have also been reported (12-14). However, such uncharged species are not easy to study due to spectral overlap with the strong absorption bands of lycopene itself.

Nevertheless, for several carotenoids the neutral radicals have been shown not to react with oxygen in an efficient manner (13, 14) (most work has concerned the model carotenoid 7,7' dihydro-ß-carotene because of its favourable spectroscopic properties): this important result shows that pro-oxidative chain reactions involving lycopene radicals are unlikely.

In summary, an overall scheme for the interaction of amino acid radicals (tryptophan) with lycopene and the lack of reactivity with oxygen is shown below (in this scheme we use LH for lycopene to clarify the hydrogen atom transfer product). The direction of the reaction involving tryptophan depending on the pH:

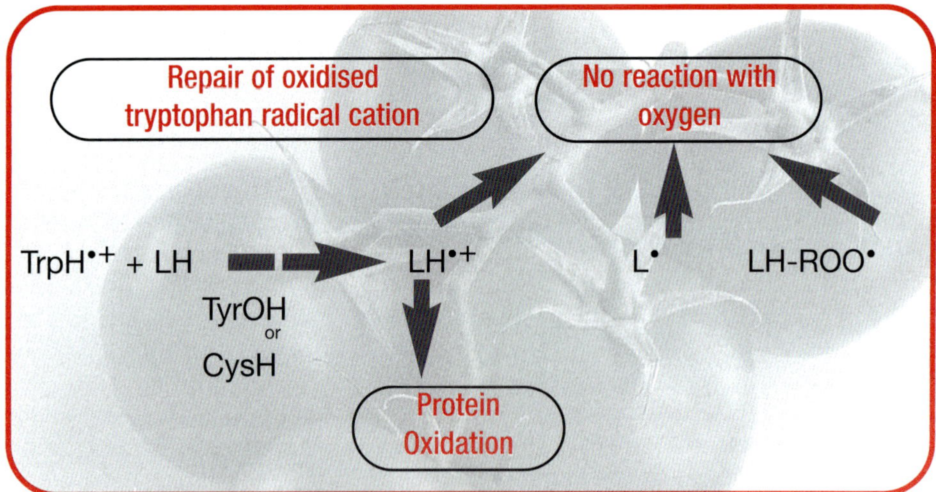

Fig 5: Scheme showing the interactions of lycopene and lycopene radicals with amino acids and oxygen

III. SINGLET OXYGEN

There have been many studies of the high efficiency with which all dietary carotenoids quench the (damaging) species called 'singlet oxygen'. Early work in mixed solvent systems suggested lycopene was markedly more efficient than ß-carotene and other carotenoids in such quenching processes. However, more recent work in a range of more biologically relevant environments shows that lycopene and ß-carotene are equally efficient as singlet oxygen quenchers. Table 2 gives typical results in DPPC unilamellar liposomes (14, 15).

Carotenoid	$K_q/10^8\ M^{-1}\ s^{-1}$
L	24.0
ß-Car	23.0
Can	23.0
Asta	5.9
Zea	2.3
ß-Crpt	1.8
Lut	1.1

Table 2: Singlet oxygen quenching rate constants for a variety of carotenoids incorporated into unilamellar DPPC liposomes

Other results by these workers show, perhaps surprisingly, little effect on the efficiency of singlet oxygen quenching when the singlet oxygen is generated inside or outside the membrane – this suggests the rate controlling step is the rate of migration of the singlet oxygen once in the membrane.

Recently Stahl and Sies (16) have shown that lycopene can act as a sunscreen via singlet oxygen quenching reactions and this suggests that lycopene supplementation could be useful in reducing skin ageing and possibly malignant melanoma. Lycopene, acting as a sunscreen from 'the inside out', may be particularly beneficial to women whose skin tends to have a higher fat level than that of men. As pointed out by these workers most of the erythemal dose (typically 65%) is encountered under non-vacation conditions when little or no sunscreen is applied so that nutritional protection could be very worthwhile. If the skin is not protected the UVA and UVB can induce the production of collagenase enzymes which accelerate the breakdown of collagen fibres and hence alter the dermal structure. This leads to loss of rigidity and elasticity in the skin. Ingestion of tomato paste, equivalent to 16 mg/day lycopene for 10 weeks was studied. After week 4 there was no significant protection against UV-induced erythema but at week 10 a significant protection was observed. Of course, ß-carotene has been used for many years to ameliorate the skin photo-sensitivity associated with the hereditary disease of erythropoetic protoporphyria and this protection is thought to be due to both the prevention of formation of singlet oxygen (by quenching the singlet oxygen precursor, the triplet state of protoporphyrin) and by direct quenching of any singlet oxygen that is formed. It seems likely that lycopene can play the same role in skin photo protection.

IV. CONCLUSIONS

Lycopene has a chemical structure with different features from all other dietary carotenoids, and it is the easiest carotenoid to oxidise and is therefore the most efficient carotenoid anti-oxidant.

Lycopene can repair (recycle) the radicals of zeaxanthin and lutein back to 'parent' zeaxanthin and lutein and this may explain the benefits of serum lycopene in reducing the onset of age-related blindness (zeaxanthin and lutein accumulate in the macular of the eye).

Lycopene like all dietary carotenoids can be beneficial to man by removing potentially damaging, strongly oxidising free radicals. However, like all other dietary carotenoids, lycopene itself is then converted to its radical cation and this can lead to deleterious effects, e.g. oxidise proteins.

Lycopene$^{\bullet+}$ is recycled to lycopene by vitamin C and hence the combination of lycopene and vitamin C may be the best dietary antioxidant system.

Lycopene, like ß-carotene, is an extremely efficient quencher of singlet oxygen in biological environments, and this may well be related to the beneficial role of lycopene in the eye and the skin.

ACKNOWLEDGEMENTS:

The authors thank Prof. F Boehm and Drs. Burke, Cantrell, El-Agamey, Land and McGarvey for much valuable collaboration.

REFERENCES:

1. Giovannucci E, Clinton SK. Tomatoes, lycopene and cancer. Proc. Soc. Exp. Biol. Med., 1998, 218, 129-139.
2. Kucuk O, Sarkar FH, Sakr W, Djuric Z et al. Phase II Randomized Clinical Trial of Lycopene Supplementation before Radical Prostatectomy. Cancer Epid. Biomarkers & Prevention, 2001, 10 861-868.
3. Kohlmeir L, Kark JD, Gomez-Garcia E, Martin BC et al. Lycopene and Myocardial Infarction Risk in the EURAMIC Study. Amer. J. Epidemiol., 1997, 146, 618-626.
4. Marles JA, Carotenoids and Eye Disease: Epidemiological Evidence. In Carotenoids in Human Health (eds. Krinsky N, Mayne ST, Seis H) New York, Marcel Dekker, p 427 — 472, 2004.
5. Gerster H, The potential role of lycopene for human health. J. Amer. College Nutr. 1997, 16, 109-126.
6. Stahl W, Sies H. Uptake of Lycopene and its Geometric Isomers is Greater from Heat-Processed Tomatoes than Unprocessed Tomato Juice in Humans. J. Nutr., 1982, 122, 2161-2166.
7. Nguyen M, Schwartz SJ. Lycopene: Chemical and biological properties. Food Technol., 1999, 53, 38-45.
8. Bertram JS. Induction of Connexin 43 by Carotenoids: Functional Consequences. Arch. Biochem. Biophys., 2004, 430, 120-126.
9. Omenn GS, Goodmen GE, Thornquist MD, Balmes J. et al. Effects of a Combination of β-carotene and vitamin A on Lung Cancer and Cardiovascular Disease.N Engl. J. Med., 1996, 334, 1150-1155.

10. Bensasson RV, Land EJ, Truscott TG. Excited States and Free Radicals in Biology and Medicine. Oxford Univ. Press, p 1-425. Oxford University Press 1993, 1-43l.
11. Burke M, Edge R, Böhm F, Truscott TG. Dietary uptake of lycopene protects human cells from singlet oxygen and nitrogen dioxide – ROS components from cigarette smoke. J. Photochem.Photobiol. B: Biol., 2001, 64, 176-178.
12. Hill T J, Land EJ, McGarvey DJ, Schalch W, Tinkler JH, Truscott TG. Interactions between Carotenoids and the $CCl_3O_2^{\bullet}$ Radical. J. Amer. Chem.Soc., 1995; 117: 8322-8326.
13. El-Agamey A, McGarvey DJ. Evidence for a Lack of Reactivity of Carotenoid Addition Radicals towards Oxygen: A Laser Flash Photolysis Study of the Reactions of Carotenoids with Acylperoxyl Radicals in Polar and Non-polar Solvents. J. Amer. Chem. Soc., 2003, 125, 3330-3340.
14. El-Agamey A, Cantrell A, Land EJ, McGarvey DJ, Truscott TG. Are dietary carotenoids beneficial? Reactions of carotenoids with oxy-radicals and singlet oxygen. Photochem. Photobiol. Sci., 2004, 3, 802-811.
15. Cantrell A, McGarvey DJ, Truscott TG, Rancan F, Boehm F. Singlet oxygen quenching by dietary carotenoids in a model membrane environment. Arch. Biochem. Biophys., 2003, 412, 47-54.
16. Sies H, Stahl W. Nutritional Protection Against Skin Damage from Sunlight. Annu. Rev. Nutr., 2004, 24, 173-200.

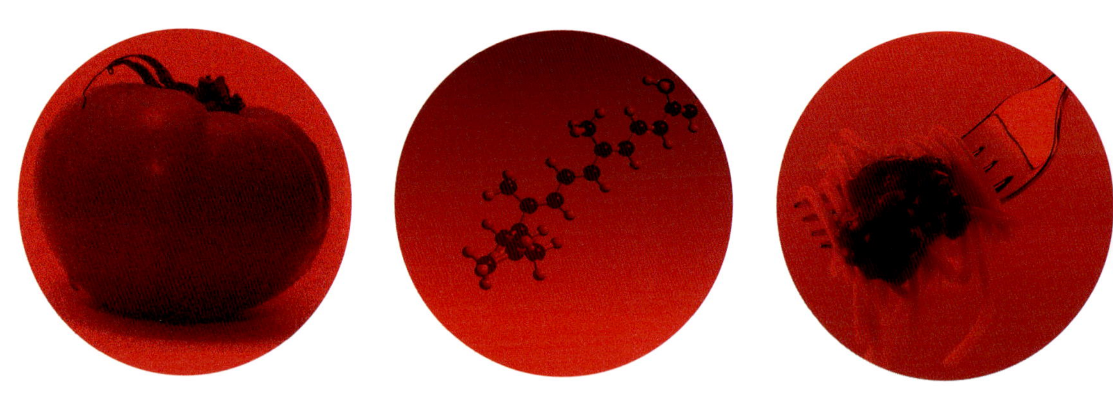

Preventing DNA Damage with Tomato Lycopene

Dr. Marissa Porrini
Dr. Patrizia Riso
Department of Food Science and Microbiology,
Division of Human Nutrition,
University of Milan,Italy

Abstract

The intake of tomato/lycopene has been suggested to reduce the risk of cancer development. Oxidative DNA lesions seem to be involved in the pathogenesis of cancer and other chronic diseases, thus the analysis of DNA damage as a biomarker of cell protection has been suggested. Several human intervention studies have been conducted in the last decade in order to verify the impact of increasing tomato lycopene intake on prevention of oxidative DNA damage. The results obtained, even if not always conclusive, seem to support the efficacy of tomato consumption and the involvement of different compounds apart from and in addition to lycopene, in the protection observed. Intervention studies on patients have also been performed with the intention/purpose of investigating the potential of using of lycopene as a chemopreventive agent. In this chapter the main results on DNA protection from oxidative damage in healthy subjects and patients on a diet enriched with tomato/lycopene are critically reviewed.

PREMISE

One of the most exciting hypotheses on the potential role of tomato products in disease prevention is that they could improve protection from DNA oxidative damage. It is widely recognised that DNA integrity is fundamental for health maintenance and, reducing the risk of cancer development. Numerous reactive species (different oxygen radicals, peroxyl radicals, aldeydes, metals etc.) that are normally produced within the body or induced by external factors, can cause alteration to the natural structure of the DNA by generating a wide variety of modified bases and lesions.

Genome instability caused by the numerous DNA damaging agents could have catastrophic effects without an efficient DNA repair enzyme system and/or the activation of signals involved in the promotion of apoptosis in irretrievably damaged cells.

The literature relevant to supporting the role of tomato/lycopene as an important anti-genotoxic food/component is steadily increasing. The specific compounds responsible for the protection afforded by tomatoes and derivatives has not been clearly demonstrated, even if lycopene has been generally mainly addressed. Tomatoes are not the only sources of this carotenoid but can also provide many different substances which may be involved in the improvement of human health. Recent research demonstrates that eating tomato products regularly increases plasma levels of different carotenoids (e.g. lycopene, ß-carotene, phytoene, phytofluene), flavonoids (e.g. rutin, naringenin, chlorogenic acid) and also vitamins (e.g. vitamin C) (1-4). A few reports (1,2, 5-7) showed an increase of several of these compounds in specific cells (lymphocytes, buccal mucosal cells, lung cells, prostate tissue). Nothing is known on the bioavailability of other different compounds, such as folates or minerals, and the effect of the whole pool of substances provided by tomato on the complex balance of active substances working in the human body.

As regards tomato lycopene, data reported in literature on its role in the prevention of DNA damage are still insufficient to make definitive conclusions. This review is intended to show and discuss the main published findings from *in vivo* studies.

EVALUATION OF DNA DAMAGE

DNA damage is generally recognized as a biomarker of "cancer risk". Particularly, continuous oxidative damage to DNA is considered a significant contributor to the age-related development of several cancers (8-10), even if a causal relationship in humans has not yet been clearly demonstrated (11, 12).

Despite the various methodological problems, data available suggest that rates and levels of oxidative DNA damage in the human body are biologically significant (13). DNA oxidative damage determines the formation of oxidized purines and pyrimidines, alkali labile sites and strand breaks (12).

Two main methods for the analysis of DNA damage are available in the literature, 1.the determination of oxidized bases by HPLC, GCMS or MSMS and, 2. the measurement of the amount of single strand breaks + alkali sensitive sites by the comet assay (with or without enzymes). However, other methods are available, such as those involving 32P post labeling and immunological techniques.

Apparently, the most abundant oxidative product of DNA bases is the 7-hydroxy-8-oxo-2'-deoxyguanosine (8-oxodG) derivative (12). It can be detected in urine, plasma and cells or tissues. This biomarker of DNA oxidation is widely used in epidemiologic and experimental studies. However inter-laboratory trials demonstrated an enormous variability in the results obtained using of different chromatographic approaches (HPLC coupled with amperometric or coulometric detection, LC-MS-MS or GC-MS). Furthermore, over-estimation is possible due to artifacts arising from DNA extraction procedures and subsequent analysis (14).

The comet assay or single cell gel electrophoresis (SCGE) technique is a reliable and sensitive method that enables the determination of DNA single strand breaks at low levels of damage (15). With this procedure, cells embedded in agarose are analyzed and then subjected to an electrophoresis step that allows the unwinding and migration of the damaged part of DNA. that The damaged fragment is recognised, when stained with ethidium bromide, as a fluorescent tail migrating from the core or head (comet). Moreover, the incubation with lesion-specific repair endonuclease allows the recognition of oxidized pyrimidines (endonuclease III) and purines (formamidopyrimidine glycosylase [FPG]) (16).

In addition, the comet assay can be used to measure cell resistance to an oxidative stress. In this case the procedure is performed on control cells and on cells that are exposed *ex vivo* to oxidant species, such as hydrogen peroxide and iron ions, or to radiations. This application can give useful information when two different conditions are compared (e.g. before and after a dietary intervention or supplementation).

Elaboration of DNA damage in the comet assay can be performed by an image analysis system (able to evaluate fluorescence intensity in the head and tail of the comets) and expressed as % DNA in tail, or alternatively the visual scoring is used (each comet is classified within a class from 0 to 4 depending on the degree of the tail observed).

It should be also noted that DNA breaks (due to both an endogenous or exogenous process) occurring in cells, can be repaired through strand break rejoining and base excision repair when cells are appropriately incubated: this normally happens *in vivo*. The comet assay including DNA digestion with endonuclease has been successfully used to evaluate DNA repair capacity (17). Another method to study repair capacity is the evaluation of the modulation of repair enzymes at different levels: the transcription of DNA repair genes (through mRNA determinations), the actual protein concentration or the enzyme activity (18).

In dietary intervention studies with tomato/ lycopene, DNA damage is generally evaluated through quantifying oxidized bases by chromatographic techniques or through the comet assay.

DIETARY LYCOPENE AND DNA DAMAGE

There is some concern about a general link between dietary antioxidant levels in blood and protection against DNA damage (19-21). This should give support to the hypothesis that components of fruit and vegetables may help to protect against cancer by decreasing endogenous DNA damage.

In this context, the results by Dusinska et al (22) are interesting as they analyzed the concentrations of different antioxidants and the relative lymphocyte endogenous DNA damage in a group of middle-aged male volunteers every month for one year. They found a significant and inverse correlation between lycopene plasma concentrations and different indicators of endogenous DNA damage; particularly strand breaks, strand breaks + FPG-sensitive sites and strand breaks + endo III-sensitive sites. The same was observed for vitamin C, while tocopherols showed a relationship with only some of the measurements considered.

On the contrary, no correspondence was observed in a previous study (23) between 8-oxodG levels and dietary antioxidant concentrations in blood of people from five European countries. The difference in the results obtained may be due to the different markers considered or to a higher heterogeneity of the populations analyzed.

INTERVENTION STUDIES WITH TOMATO/ LYCOPENE AND DNA DAMAGE

Intervention studies represent a unique tool for the demonstration of the "functional and protective" properties of foods or their components. Unfortunately they are often expensive, time consuming and, above all, need to be well designed in order to take into the right consideration the confounding factors related with individual eating habits. Furthermore, compliance with the diet can be low, and consequently subjects have to be well motivated and instructed.

Controlled human dietary interventions concerning the specific effects of tomato/lycopene intake on oxidative DNA damage in humans are scarce. Data can be distinguished on the basis of the type of intervention (tomato products, tomato extracts, supplements) or the subjects involved (healthy vs. patients).
In this review, data in literature will be presented distinguishing between intervention studies carried out with healthy subjects (Tables 1 and 2) and with patients (Table 3).

INTERVENTION STUDIES WITH HEALTHY SUBJECTS

The first published intervention trials with tomato products had rather inadequate study design. However, their results aroused great interest in the scientific community.

The first one is that of Pool-Zobel et al (24) who found that the consumption of 330 ml of tomato juice (40 mg lycopene) and also carrot juice (22.3 mg lycopene, 15.7 mg α-carotene) for one week was able to significantly decrease endogenous levels of strand breaks in lymphocyte DNA evaluated by the comet assay. Dried spinach powder (10 g; 11.3 mg lutein) did not have the same impact. On the contrary, oxidative base damage determined after the digestion step with endonucleases was not modified by tomato intervention. Despite these interesting and stimulating results, the study has been criticised because of its lack of a wash-out period between dietary interventions. The same group also investigated the potential mechanisms by which the vegetables used in the study could reduce DNA damage, hypothesizing an effect of modulation on expression of cytosolic GSTP1 and DNA repair enzymes (25).

Rao et al (26) also suggested a possible role of tomato consumption in cell protection; they found a trend towards a decrease in lymphocyte 8-oxodG (not significant) following the intake of different tomato products (540 ml tomato juice, 126 g spaghetti sauce and 1.2-2.5 g tomato oleoresin) providing from 20.5 to 150 mg lycopene for one week. Indeed, a decrease (even if not significant) in another oxidized base (8-hydroxyguanine) was found in lymphocytes of volunteers eating a single portion of 360 -728 g tomato (8g/Kg body mass) (27). The highest decrease in 8-hydroxyguanine after the tomato intake was observed in those subjects with high basal levels of DNA damage; however, total base damage did not change, mostly due to an increase in 8-hydroxyadenine. Despite the limits of this study, the fact that the intake of a single portion of tomato can enhance cell defence supports the concept of a *day by day* contribution of vegetables to the overall protection. However, these preliminary data need a confirmation through a controlled experimental protocol and the evaluation of biomarkers of DNA damage by means of other chromatographic techniques different from to the GC/MS method used by the authors. In this regard, more recently Boyle et al (28) employed a two-phase crossover design in order to evaluate the effect of a single meal rich in flavonoids consisting of onion or onion + cherry tomatoes on antioxidant levels and different biomarkers of oxidative stress. Following the onion meal, both endogenous base oxidation and H_2O_2-induced DNA damage in lymphocytes (evaluated by means of comet assay) were significantly reduced 4-8 hours after the intake. A significant decrease in the urinary excretion of 8-oxodG (evaluated by means of an immunoassay) was also observed. The onion + cherry tomatoes meal only decreased endogenous pyrimidine oxidation. The authors concluded that the combined meal was less effective than the onion meal hypothesizing a competing effect between flavonoids and other nutrients.

In order to evaluate the protective effect against DNA damage, we have also performed several intervention studies with different tomato products on healthy young volunteers (Table 2) in order to evaluate the protective effect against DNA damage. From the first repeated measure cross-over design we found that the daily consumption of 60 g tomato puree (about 16 mg lycopene) for 21 days increased lymphocyte protection from H_2O_2-induced DNA damage evaluated by the comet assay (29). In a later study, it was possible to confirm this effect also after the intake of 25 g tomato puree (about 7 mg lycopene) for two weeks, even if, in this study, the absence of a control group may be considered a potential bias (30). Interestingly, in our studies, we found for the first time an inverse and significant correlation between plasma and lymphocyte lycopene concentration and DNA damage. The intake of the same amount of tomato puree (25 g, 7 mg lycopene) added to spinach (150 g, 9 mg lutein, 4 mg ß-carotene) did not increase the protection as expected. The correlation analysis performed on lymphocyte carotenoid concentrations vs. DNA damage demonstrated that neither lutein nor lycopene could be uniquely responsible for the protection observed (31). However, an interesting point emerged: in a long term condition of carotenoid deprivation diet, just the regular addition of one vegetable rich in antioxidants can improve DNA protection possibly modulating "one factor" of the equilibrium of the very complex antioxidant system.

The results obtained in our latest studies confirmed that a wide antioxidant network including both water- and fat-soluble compounds, not completely identified, is probably involved in cell protection. Particularly, the daily intake of different tomato products (raw tomato, tomato sauce and puree) for three weeks, providing about 8 mg lycopene, 1 mg ß-carotene and 11 mg/day vitamin C on average, resulted in a significant increase in lymphocyte lycopene and, above all, vitamin C concentrations paralleled by an improvement in DNA protection (1). More recently, in a controlled double blind cross-over repeated measure design we demonstrated that the intake of 250 ml of a tomato drink providing about 6 mg lycopene, 1 mg ß-carotene, 3 mg phytoene, 4 mg phytofluene and 1.8 mg α-tocopherol for 26 days increased lymphocyte resistance to DNA oxidative damage and determined also the enhancement in lymphocytes of all the carotenoids present in the drink (2). In this regard, the study by Briviba et al (32) should be mentioned as they did not find a significant protective effect, on both smokers and non smokers, after the regular intake for two weeks of a tomato oleoresin providing the same compounds in different amounts (4.9 mg lycopene, 0.5 mg phytoene, 0.4 mg phytofluene, 1.2 mg α-tocopherol) for two weeks. The authors found only a significant increase in the number of comets in class 0 (correspondent to undamaged DNA), and concluded that a tendency to reduce endogenous DNA strand breaks was observed after the intake of the tomato oleoresin. In our opinion the lack of significance of DNA damage evaluated by the authors with respect to our data can be due to the biomarker of DNA damage considered. In fact, endogenous DNA damage is extremely low compared to H_2O_2-induced DNA damage (less than 5% vs. more than 50% depending on the H_2O_2 dose) and generally rather homogeneous in healthy subjects. When considering endogenous DNA damage the use of lesion-specific repair endonuclease could be advantageous allowing the determination of both SSBs and oxidized bases as previously discussed.

In summary, the data considered suggest that lycopene might be a marker of a cell's increased protection towards DNA damage more than the *actual* main compound responsible for such an action. This may partially explain some results from other researchers who used lycopene supplements instead of whole foods. Astley et al (33), for example, did not find any effect on single strand breaks in oxidized or control peripheral blood lymphocytes after the intake of 15 mg/d lycopene for four weeks in healthy male volunteers. In contrast, Tobergsen and Collins (34) found a positive effect of pure lycopene supplementation on lymphocyte DNA repair. They hypothesized that the result was simply due to an antioxidant effect against atmospheric oxygen action rather than a modulation of repair, in contrast to what was suggested by Pool-Zobel et al (25).

Another interesting study is that of Arab et al (6) who evaluated in a randomized clinical trial the effect of the supplementation for two weeks with a carotenoid-rich vegetable (containing 23 mg lycopene and other carotenoids) and a supplement of vitamin C and α-tocopherol (250 mg and 50 IU respectively) or a placebo treatment on carotenoid levels and DNA damage. DNA damage was measured in peripheral blood leukocytes and in lung epithelial cells (by comet assay) of subjects exposed to ambient air or to 0.4 ppm ozone while exercising intermittently for two hours in a Plexiglas and steel chamber.

DNA damage in lung epithelial cells significantly increased in subjects on placebo treatment after ozone exposure, while remained constant in those receiving the supplementation. On the contrary, leukocyte DNA damage was not different after ozone or antioxidant supplementation, probably suggesting that this type of cell is not specifically affected by the oxidant used even if further confirmation is necessary.

From these and other studies, another consideration comes out: the intake of tomato/lycopene seems to protect cell DNA *ex vivo* not only from different oxidative species such as H_2O_2 (29), Fe^{2+} (1), ozone (6) but also UV radiation (unpublished data from our group). Moreover, the same a protective activity was observed against other species such as $CCl_3O_2^{\bullet}$ (35), $NO_2^{\bullet}$ (36), singlet oxygen (37) even if, in these studies, this was not specifically associated to with the evaluation of DNA damage.

INTERVENTION STUDIES WITH PATIENTS

There are only a few interesting studies in the literature evaluating whether lycopene may be useful in the prevention or control of specific cancers. Epidemiologic data support the idea that a consistently lower risk of cancer for a variety of anatomic sites is associated with higher consumption of tomatoes and tomato-based products. The evidence for a benefit was demonstrated to be strongest for cancers of the prostate, lung and stomach (38).

Moreover, the presence of relatively high amounts of lycopene in the prostate raises the question of a potential specific activity of the substance in this kind of tissue protection. The prostate, in fact, is particularly vulnerable to oxidative attack, cell turnover is very fast and the levels of DNA repair enzymes are lower with respect to other tissues (7).

Based on this body of evidence, a number of preliminary studies have been conducted in order to probe the possibility of using tomato/lycopene as a chemopreventive agent.

The first recognised report is that of Kukuk et al (39,40) who, in a randomized, two-arm intervention study, supplemented the diet of a small group of men with newly diagnosed prostate cancer, with a tomato oleoresin extract providing 30 mg lycopene/day for 3 weeks before radical prostatectomy. Results were compared to those of a control group whose diet was not supplemented. DNA damage in lymphocytes assessed by measuring the oxidized base 5-hydroxy-methyl-deoxyuridine (5-OH-mdU) did not change after the intervention. Furthermore, only some of the subjects had an increase in plasma lycopene concentration. Despite these results, subjects in the intervention group had smaller and more confined tumors, suggesting a potential beneficial effect of tomato extract. Changes in other clinical parameters were also observed: an 18% decrease in PSA levels, an increase in connexin 43 protein level, a decrease in IGF-1 and IGFBP-3 levels but no apparent effect on bcl-2 and bax proteins.

Data reported by Chen et al (41) and Bowen et al (7) are also interesting. They carried out a randomized placebo-controlled study on thirty-two patients with localized prostate adenocarcinoma. Subjects were asked to consume tomato sauce-based pasta dishes for 3 weeks (30 mg lycopene/day) before radical prostatectomy. Different markers were analyzed. Particularly interesting was the significant uptake of lycopene into the prostate tissue and the decrease in DNA damage (evaluated as 8-oxodG) both in leukocytes and prostate after the dietary treatment. Moreover, a reduction in PSA levels and an increase in apoptotic cell death in benign prostate hyperplasia was also observed (42). All these data provide *in vivo* evidence that tomato sauce consumption may contribute to suppress the progression of prostate cancer. However, due to the small number of subjects involved in these intervention studies, further data are necessary to confirm the protective action observed and to exclude any adverse effect. To this end several clinical trials are in progress.

REMARKS AND PERSPECTIVE

On the whole, the data reviewed seem to support a protective effect of tomato consumption against cell DNA damage.
The evaluation of biomarkers of DNA damage (e.g. SSBs, oxidized bases) in target cells can be used to predict the impact of specific foods on disease prevention. However, the evaluation of DNA damage is extremely difficult so that standardized and validated procedures are needed to achieve reliable data. With this goal, much work has been carried out by the European Standards Committee on Oxidative DNA Damage (ESCODD) (14). Particularly sources of artefacts have been identified and standard protocols developed in order to minimize DNA oxidation during sample preparation. The accuracy of measurement obtained by different chromatographic techniques and the enzymic approach have been compared. However, further efforts are still needed. (14).

Another important goal is that of carefully performing a statistically relevant number of controlled dietary intervention studies. These would support the bulk of epidemiologic evidence on the protective effect of fruit and vegetables consumption against disease risk but not yet confirmed by supplementation with pure compounds (43, 44).

Complex matrices such as vegetables contain, in fact, numerous different compounds which can act in a concerted manner providing active protection. In this context, the interaction between compounds present in tomatoes and in other vegetables would seem to be an interesting but insufficiently studied topic.

Regarding the special case of lycopene, recent research on animal models and/or cell culture studies (not considered in this review) have provided important contributions to the understanding of its potential mechanisms of action. Mechanisms such as those involved in apoptosis and cell growth regulation may be exploited in the future to limit the progression of cancer cells.

Finally, in view of the hypothesis that a “genetic” component could characterize a vulnerable population, more should be done to understand the genetic susceptibility to DNA damage and repair. For example it is crucial to establish the role of different polymorphs of repairing enzymes or other components of the endogenous defence system on the individual response to the exposure to dietary factors such those provided by the tomato. To this regard it was recently hypothesized that differences in Base Excision Repair capacity (such as those potentially related to polymorphisms in the XRCC1 gene) could modulate the effect of dietary antioxidant intake on prostate cancer risk (45). In this pilot case-control study it was found that prostate cancer risk was highest among men who were homozygous for the common allele at the XRCC1 codon 399 and had low dietary intake of vitamin E (OR=2.4; 95%CI, 1.0-5.6) or lycopene (OR=2.0; 95%CI, 0.8-4.9). On the contrary a low intake of these antioxidants in men without this genotype hardly increased prostate cancer risk.

If such observations are confirmed in the future much could be known not only about individual predisposition to "disease risk", but also about the real potential of a specific dietary intervention as "simple" preventive approach.

Dietary intervention	Carotenoids provided	Biomarker	Target cell
330 ml tomato juice 330 ml carrot juice 10 g dried spinach 1 week	40 mg lycopene 22.3 mg β-carotene + 15.7 mg α-carotene 11.3 mg lutein	SSBs and oxidized bases by comet assay	lymphocyte
540 ml tomato juice 126 g spaghetti sauce 1.2-2.5 g oleoresin 1 week	50.4 mg lycopene 20.5-39.2 mg lycopene 75-150 mg lycopene	8-oxodG by HPLC, electrochemical detector	lymphocyte
360-728 g tomato single portion	Not reported	8—OH guanine and other oxidized bases by GC-MS	white blood cells
Tomato oleoresin extract capsules 3 per day 2 weeks	4.9 mg lycopene 0.5 mg phytoene 0.4 mg phytofluene 1.2 mg α-tocopherol	SSBs by comet assay	lymphocyte
Carotenoid-rich vegetable juice 2 weeks	23 mg lycopene 2 mg α-carotene 0.7 mg β-carotene 0.4 mg lutein 0.1 mg zeaxanthin	SSBs and oxidized bases by comet assay	lung epithelial cells, leukocytes
Fried onions or fried onions + fresh cherry tomatoes One meal	Flavonoids flavonoids + carotenoids	Endogenous and H_2O_2-induced damage by comet assay 8-oxodG by immunoassay	lymphocyte
Supplements 1 week	15 mg lycopene 15 mg β-carotene 15 mg lutein	SSBs and oxidized bases by comet assay	lymphocyte
34 Natural isolate capsules 4 weeks	15 mg lycopene 15 mg lutein 15 mg β-carotene	SSBs by comet assay	lymphocyte

Table1: Modulation of DNA damage by tomato/lycopene evaluated in intervention studies with healthy subjects

Main results	Ref
Decreased SSBs were observed after the three interventions with a minor effect of spinach. Only carrot juice reduced oxydized pyrimidine. No food improved protection against H_2O_2. Increased cytosolic proteins GSTP1 and DNA repair proteins were observed in a subset of individuals	24
All the tomato products reduced 8-oxodG in lymphocytes (not significant)	25
Falls of 8 —hydroxyguanine (not significant) were registered in those subjects with high basal DNA damage. Total base damage was unchanged	27
Tendency to reduce endogenous DNA strand breaks in non-smokers (32%) and smokers (39%). Increased comets in class 0 (undamaged DNA) after the intervention	32
Lower DNA damage in lung epithelial cells after exposition to ozone. No effect on lymphocyte DNA damage	6
The onion meal was effective in reducing DNA damage. The combined meal affected endogenous base oxidation but not H_2O_2-induced DNA damage in lymphocytes. No effect on urine excretion of 8-oxodG	28
Supplementation increased DNA repair (lower DNA damage) in subjects who showed increase in lycopene concentration. No specific effect was observed for lutein	34
No effect of lycopene and lutein but β-carotene on lymphocyte DNA damage (SSB) in control cells	33

Table1: Modulation of DNA damage by tomato/lycopene evaluated in intervention studies with healthy subjects

Tomato intervention	Lycopene intake (main other antioxidants) mg/day	DNA protection (oxidant used)	Other results	Ref
60 g puree 3 wks	16 mg	+ 30-40% (H_2O_2)	Lycopene concentration increased by 185% after tomato intake. Inverse significant correlation between lycopene level and DNA damage (r=-0.8, P<0.01)	29
25 g puree 2 wks	7 mg	7 mg+50% (H_2O_2)	Lycopene concentration increased both in plasma and lymphocytes (+ 323% and 81%). The inverse correlation between lycopene level and DNA damage was confirmed (r=-0.8, P<0.0001)	30
25 g paste + 100g spinach 3 wks	7 mg (9 mg lutein, 4 mg β-carotene)	+30-50% (H_2O_2)	Lycopene but also lutein concentration increased by 940% and 150% in plasma and by 600% and 192% in lymphocytes. An inverse correlation between lymphocyte lycopene but not lutein concentrations and DNA damage was registered (r=-0.6, P<0.001)	31
15 g paste, 100 g raw, 60 g sauce 3 wks	8 mg (11 mg vitamin C)	+ 24% (Fe^{2+})	Lycopene concentration increased both in plasma and lymphocytes (+ 53% and +70 %). A significant increase of vitamin C was registered (plasma: +35% lymphocytes:+236%).	1
250 ml Lyc-o-Mato drink 26 days	5.7 mg (3.7 mg phytoene, 2.7 mg phytofluene, 1 mg β-carotene, 1.8 mg α-tocopherol)	+ 42 % (H_2O_2)	All the carotenoid provided increased both in plasma and lymphocytes: Lycopene increased by 68% and 105% Phytoene by 92% and 159% Phytofluene by 61% and 84% β-carotene by 28% and 51% Data suggested the involvement of different compounds in DNA protection	2

Table2: Modulation of DNA damage by tomato/lycopene evaluated in intervention studies with healthy subjects

Pathology	Type of intervention	Carotenoids provided	Biomarker	Target cell	Main results	Ref
Prostate	Tomato oleoresin capsules 3 weeks	30 mg lycopene	5-OH-mdU by GC-MS	lymphocyte	Smaller tumors in supplemented subjects with respect to control group but no effect on the DNA oxidation product considered.	39, 40
Prostate	Tomato sauce-based pasta 3 weeks	30 mg lycopene	8-OHdG by HPLC-EC	leukocyte	Prostate-21.3% 8-OHdG/10^5dG in leukocyte -28.3% 8-OHdG/10^5dG in prostate tissue	7, 41

Table 3: Modulation of DNA damage by tomato/lycopene evaluated in intervention studies with patients

REFERENCES:

1. Riso P, Visioli F, Erba D, Testolin G, Porrini M. Lycopene and vitamin C concentrations increase in plasma and lymphocytes after tomato intake. Effects on cellular antioxidant protection. Eur J Clin Nutr. 2004; 58: 1350-1358.
2. Porrini M, Riso P, Brusamolino A, Berti C, Guarnieri S, Visioli F. Daily intake of a formulated tomato drink affects carotenoid plasma and lymphocyte concentrations and improves cellular antioxidant protection. Br J Nutr 2005; 93:93—99.
3. Simonetti P, Gardana C, Riso P, Mauri PL, Pietta PG, Porrini M. Glycosylated flavonoids from tomato puree are bioavailable in humans. Nutr Res 2005; 25:717-726.
4. Bugianesi R, Salucci M, Leonardi C, Ferracane R, Catasta G, Azzini E, Maiani G. Effect of domestic cooking on human bioavailability of naringenin, chlorogenic acid, lycopene and beta-carotene in cherry tomatoes. Eur J Nutr. 2004 ; 43(6) :360-366.
5. Reifen R, Haftel L, Faulks R, Southon S, Kaplan I, Schwarz B. Plasma and buccal mucosal cell response to short-term supplementation with all-trans beta-carotene and lycopene in human volunteers. Int J Mol Med 2003; 12(6):989-993.
6. Arab L, Steck-Scott S, Fleishauer AT. Lycopene and the lung. Exp Biol Med 2002; 227:894-899.

7. Bowen P, Chen L, Stacewicz-Sapuntzakis M, Duncan C, Sharifi R, Ghosh L, Kim H-S, Christov-Tzelkov K, van Breemen R. Tomato sauce supplementation and prostate cancer: lycopene accumulation and modulation of biomarkers of carcinogenesis. Exp Biol Med 2002; 227:886-893.
8. Halliwell B, Gutteridge JMC. Free radicals in biology and medicine. 3rd ed. Oxford, United Kingdom: Oxford University Press 1999.
9. Totter JR. Spontaneous cancer and its possible relationship to oxygen metabolism. Proc Natl Acad Sci USA 1980; 77:1763-7.
10. Ames BN, Shigenaga MK, Hagen TM. Oxidants, antioxidants and the degenerative diseases of aging. Proc Natl Acad Sci USA 1993; 90:7915-22.
11. Halliwell B. Why and how should we measure oxidative DNA damage in nutritional studies? How far have we come? Am J Clin Nutr 2000; 72:1082-7.
12. Loft S, Poulsen H.E. Cancer risk and oxidative DNA damage in man. J Mol Med 1996;74:297-312.
13. Halliwell B. Effect of diet on cancer development: is oxidative DNA damage a biomarker? Free Rad Biol & Med 2002; 32:968-974.
14. Gedik CM, Collins A. Establishing the background level of base oxidation in human lymphocyte DNA: results of an interlaboratory validation study. FASEB J 2005;19:82-84.
15. Horváthová E, Slameňová D, Hličíková L, Mandal TK, Gábelová A, Collins A. The nature and origin of DNA single-strand breaks determined with the comet assay. Mut Res 1998; 409:163-171.
16. Collins AR, Duthie S, Dobson VL. Direct enzymic detection of endogenous oxidative base damage in human lymphocyte DNA. Carcinogenesis 1993;14:1733-5.
17. Collins AR, Ai-Guo M, Duthie SJ. The kinetics of repair of oxidative DNA damage (strand breaks and oxidized pyrimidines) in human cells. Mut Res 1995; 336:69-77.
18. Moller P, Loft S. Interventions with antioxidants and nutrients in relation to oxidative DNA damage and repair. Mut Res 2004; 551:79-89.
19. Mooney LA, Bell DA, Santella RM et al Contribution of genetic and nutritional factors to DNA damage in heavy smokers. Carcinogenesis 1997; 18:503-9.
20. Collins AR, Olmedilla B, Southon S, Granado F, Duthie S. Serum carotenoids and oxidative DNA damage in human lymphocytes. Carcinogenesis 1998;19:2159-62.
21. Palli D, Masala G, Vineis P, Garte S, Saieva C, Krogh V, Panico S, Tumino R, Munnia A, Riboli E, Peluso M. Biomarkers of dietary intake of micronutrients modulate DNA adduct levels in healthy adults. Carcinogenesis 2003; 24:739-46.
22. Duŝinská M, Vallová B, Ursínyová M, Hladíková V, Smolková B, Wsólová L, Raŝlová K, Collins AR. DNA damage and antioxidants; fluctuations through the year in a central European population group. Food Chem Toxicol 2002; 40:1119-23.
23. Collins AR, Gedik CM, Olmedilla B, Southon S, Bellizzi M. Oxidative DNA damage measured in human lymphocytes: large differences between sexes and between countries, and correlations with heart disease mortality rates. FASEB J 1998;12:1397-1400.

24. Pool-Zobel BL, Bub A, Müller H, Wollowski I, Rechkemmer G. Consumption of vegetables reduces genetic damage in humans: first results of a human intervention trial with carotenoid-rich foods. Carcinogenesis 1997;18:1847-50.
25. Pool-Zobel BL, Bub A, Liegibel M, Treptow-van Lishaut S, Rechkemmer G. Mechanisms by which vegetable consumption reduces genetic damage in humans. Cancer Epidemiol Biomar & Prev 1998;7:891-9.
26. Rao AV, Agarwal S. Bioavailability and in vivo antioxidant properties of lycopene from tomato products and their possible role in the prevention of cancer. Nutr Cancer 1998; 31:199-203.
27. Rehman A, Bourne LC, Halliwell B, Rice-Evans CA. Tomato consumption modulates oxidative DNA damage in humans. Biochem Biophys Res Com 1999; 262:828-31.
28. Boyle SP, Dobson VL, Duthie SJ, Kyle JAM, Collins AR. Absorption and DNA protective effects of flavonoid glycosides from an onion meal. Eur J Nutr 2000; 39:213-23
29. Riso P, Pinder A, Santangelo A Porrini M. Does tomato consumption effectively increase the resistance of lymphocyte DNA to oxidative damage? Am J Clin Nutr 1999; 69:712-18.
30. Porrini M, Riso P. Lymphocyte lycopene concentration and DNA protection from oxidative damage is increased in woman after a short period of tomato consumption. J Nutr 2000; 130:189-92.
31. Porrini M, Riso P, Oriani G. Spinach and tomato consumption increases lymphocyte DNA resistance to oxidative stress but this is not related to carotenoid concentrations. Eur J Nutr. 2002; 41:95-100.
32. Briviba K, Kulling SE, Möseneder J, Watzl B, Rechkemmer G. Bub A. Effects of supplementing a low-carotenoid diet with a tomato extract for 2 weeks on endogenous levels of DNA single strand breaks and immune functions in healthy non-smokers and smokers. Carcinogenesis 2004; 25:2373-2378.
33. Astley SB, Hughes DA, Wright AJA, Elliott RM, Southon S. DNA damage and susceptibility to oxidative damage in lymphocytes: effects of carotenoids in vitro and in vivo. Br J Nutr 2004; 91:53-61.
34. Tobergsen AC, Collins AR. Recovery of human lymphocytes from oxidative DNA damage; the apparent enhancement of DNA repair by carotenoids is probably simply an antioxidant effect. Eur J Nutr 2000;39:80-5.
35. Yaping Z, Suping Q, Wenlia Y, Honga S, Sideb Y, Dapua W. Antioxidant activity of lycopene exctracted from tomato paste towards trichloromethyl peroxyl radical CCL3O2. Food Chem 2002; 77:209-211.
36. Böhm F, Edge R, Burke M, Truscott TG. Dietary uptake of lycopene protects human cells from singlet oxygen and nitrogen dioxide – ROS components from cigarette smoke. J Photochem Photobiol B: Biol 2001; 64:176-178.
37. Di Mascio P, Kaiser S, Sies H. Lycopene as the most efficient biological carotenoid singlet oxygen quencher. Arch Biochem Biophys 1989; 274:532-538.
38. Giovannucci E. Tomatoes, tomato-based products, lycopene, and cancer: review of the epidemiologic literature. J Natl Cancer Inst 1999; 91:317-31.

39. Kucuk O, Sarkar FH, Sakr W, Djuric Z, Pollak MN, Khachik F, Li Y-W, Banerjee M, Grignon D, Bertram J, Crissman JD, Pontes EJ, Wood DP Jr. Phase II randomized clinical trial of lycopene supplementation before radical prostatectomy. Cancer Epidemiol Biomarkers Prev 2001; 10:861-68.
40. Kucuk O, Sarkar FH, Djuric Z, Sakr W, Pollak MN, Khachik F, Banerjee M, Bertram JS, Wood DP. Effects of lycopene supplementation in patients with localized prostate cancer. Exp Biol Med 2002; 227: 881-885.
41. Chen L, Stacewicz-Sapuntzakis M, Duncan C, Sharifi R, Ghosh L, van Breemen R, Ashton D, Bowen PE. Oxidative DNA damage in prostate cancer patients consuming tomato sauce-based entrees as a whole-food intervention. J Natl Cancer Inst 2001; 93:1872-9.
42. Kim H-S, Bowen P, Chen L, Duncan C, Ghosh L, Sharifi R, Christov K. Effects of tomato sauce consumption on apoptotic cell death in prostate benign hyperplasia and carcinoma. Nutr Cancer 2003; 47:40-7.
43. The Alpha-Tocopherol, Beta-Carotene Cancer Prevention Study Group. The effect of vitamin E and beta-carotene on the incidence of lung cancer and other cancers in male smokers. N Eng J Med 1994; 330:1029-35.
44. Omenn GS, Goodman GE, Thornquist MD, Balmes J, Cullen MR, Glass A, Keogh JP, Meyskens F, Valaris B, Williams JH, Barnhart S, Hammer S. Effects of a combination of β-carotene and vitamin A on lung cancer and cardiovascular disease. N Eng J Med 1996; 334:1150-1155.
45. van Gils CH, Bostick RM, Stern MC, Taylor JA. Differences in base excision repair capacity may modulate the effect of dietary antioxidant intake on prostate cancer risk: an example of polymorphisms in the XRCC1 gene. Cancer Epidemiol Biomarkers Prev 2002; 11:1279-1284.

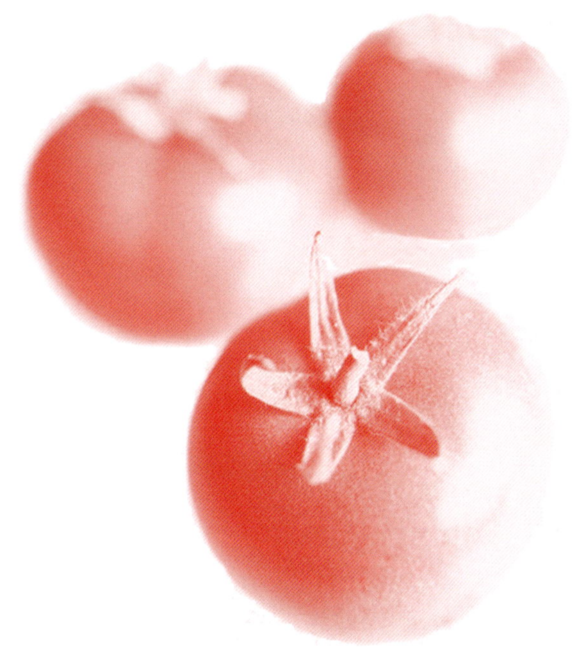

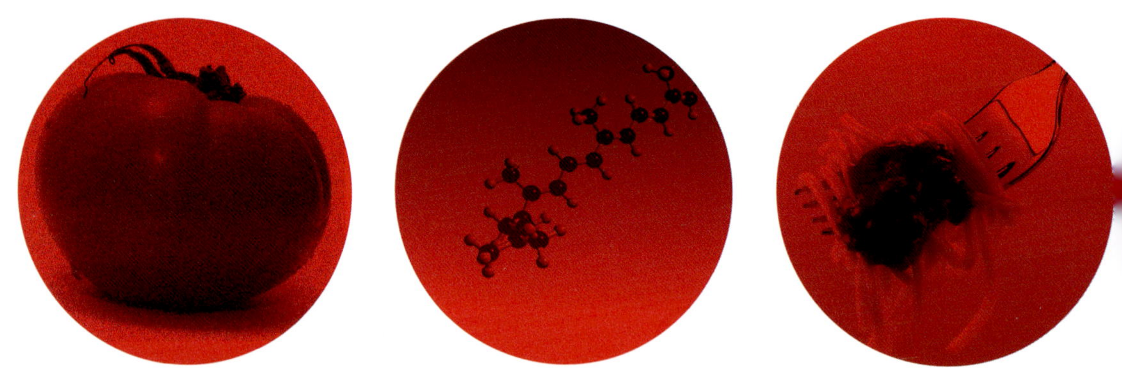

Cancer Prevention by Dietary Tomato Lycopene and its Molecular Mechanisms

Dr. Yoav Sharoni
Dr. Yossi Levy
Department of Clinical Biochemistry, Faculty of Health Sciences, Ben-Gurion University of the Negev and Soroka Medical Center of Kupat Holim, Beer-Sheva, Israel

Abstract

Carcinogenesis is a multistage process involving molecular and cellular alterations that lead to tumor initiation, promotion and progression. Successful prevention of cancer should interfere in all stages of the carcinogenic process. In this review, we suggest that lycopene can act as an initiation blocking agent by inducing a set of detoxification and antioxidant enzymes (Phase II enzymes) through the activation of the antioxidant response element (ARE) transcription system. In addition, lycopene can suppress the promotion stage by inhibiting growth factor- and hormone-induced cell proliferation. The latter effects are achieved through modulation of several cell processes such as gap junction communication and cell cycle progression. We argue, however, that these cancer preventing effects are not achieved by lycopene alone but through its combination with other tomato carotenoids, such as phytoene and phytofluene, and other phytonutrients found in various fruits and vegetables.

I. CONCEPT OF CHEMOPREVENTION

Despite the considerable efforts that have been invested into finding new methods for cancer treatment, the mortality and incidence of cancer have not substantially declined. For this reason, more emphasis is now being placed on cancer prevention. Several studies have demonstrated that environmental factors are involved as risk factors in the majority of human cancers and that a significant amount of cancer-related mortalities can be prevented by eliminating these factors from our environment or at least by avoiding exposure to them. However, obviously in practice, it is almost impossible for humans to elude daily environmental exposure to diverse carcinogens. Therefore, more effective strategies have been sought to find agents which can inhibit, delay or reverse carcinogenic processes. The term "chemoprevention," which was coined in 1976 by Sporn (1), describes the use of specific natural, synthetic, or biologic agents for this purpose. In particular, for persistent, long-term prevention of cancer, changes in diet rather than drug application is a more sensible approach.

Carcinogenesis is a multistage process that involves molecular and cellular alterations. It largely consists of three separate, but closely linked stages – tumor initiation, promotion and progression (2, 3). Initiation is defined as a mutagenic event in nature and generally results from DNA damage by physical, chemical or viral exposure. Promotion is characterized by transformation of an initiated cell into a population of preneoplastic cells as a result of epigenetic alterations in the cell by chronic exposure to tumor promoters, such as growth factors, or hormones. Progression is regarded as a final stage of carcinogenesis, in which the preneoplastic cells are converted into an invasive and metastatic cell population.

Based on this multistage carcinogenesis model, Wattenberg (4, 5) classified chemopreventive compounds into “blocking agents” or “suppressing agents.” Blocking agents are compounds which inhibit the formation of reactive carcinogens from pro-carcinogens by metabolic activation, or which prevent active carcinogens from reaching or reacting with critical cellular targets in the initiation stage of carcinogenesis. One of the plausible mechanisms by which blocking agents confer their chemopreventive activity is the induction of a set of detoxification and antioxidant enzymes through the activation of intracellular signaling mediated by nuclear transcription factor Nuclear factor E2-related factor 2 (Nrf2) (6-8).

Suppressing agents, on the other hand, inhibit the premalignant and malignant transformation of initiated cells during the stage of promotion and progression, respectively. In contrast to initiation, tumor promotion is recognized as a relatively lengthy and reversible process in which actively proliferating preneoplastic cells accumulate. Progression, the final stage of neoplastic transformation, involves the growth of a tumor with invasive and metastatic potential. Documented activities of suppressing agents include inhibition of basal and growth factor induced cell proliferation, and attenuation of hormone action in estrogen- and androgen-dependent tumors in breast and prostate cancer respectively. In addition, suppressing agents were reported to regulate cell communication by the formation of gap junctions (9) and induction of apoptosis or terminal differentiation which are important mechanisms for inhibiting tumor promotion and progression (5).

Obviously, diet can be a source of potential chemopreventive agents. In fact, alongside lycopene, a number of natural compounds with inhibitory effects on tumorogenesis have been identified in our diet. These compounds include isothiocyanates from cruciferous vegetables, catechins from green tea, resveratrol from grape seeds and red wine, curcuminoids from turmeric, procyanidins from various fruits and nuts, isoflavones from soybean, and antioxidant vitamins in various foods (10, 11).

Here we review evidence that lycopene and other carotenoids are active in cancer prevention by their blocking and suppressing activity. However, since lycopene is found in blood and tissues at low concentrations, its main activity depends on its combination with other dietary ingredients, specifically with those found in the tomato. Before analyzing the molecular mechanisms underlyng tomato lycopene activity in cancer prevention, it is important to review the epidemiological data showing the inverse correlation between lycopene and tomato product consumption and blood level and the risk of cancer.

II. THE PROTECTIVE ROLE OF LYCOPENE IN CANCER PREVENTION: EVIDENCE FROM EPIDEMIOLOGICAL AND INTERVENTION STUDIES

A comprehensive review of the epidemiological literature on the relation of tomato consumption and cancer was recently published by Giovannucci (12). He found that among 72 studies, 57 reported inverse associations between tomato intake or blood lycopene level and the risk of cancer at a defined anatomic site. 35 out of 57 of these inverse associations were statistically significant. None of the cited studies indicated that higher tomato consumption or blood lycopene level significantly increased the risk of cancer at any of the investigated sites. The evidence of a beneficial effect was strongest for cancers of the prostate, lung, and stomach. Data were also suggestive of a beneficial effect for cancers of the pancreas, colon and rectum, esophagus, oral cavity, breast, and cervix. Giovannucci suggests that although lycopene may contribute to these beneficial effects of tomato-containing foods, this has not been conclusively proven. The anticancer properties can be explained by the interactions that take place among multiple components found in tomatoes. Based on the results of epidemiological studies showing an inverse correlation between lycopene consumption and prostate cancer risk as pointed out in Giovannucci's comprehensive review, cancer of the prostate is the focus of lycopene research and several new studies have appeared in the literature. For example, an ecologic (multi-country statistical) approach has found that tomatoes reduce the risk of prostate cancer, most likely due to the action of lycopene (13). Two small-scale, preliminary intervention studies on prostate cancer patients were carried out with natural tomato preparations. In one, Bowen et al (14) showed that after dietary intervention, serum and prostate lycopene concentrations were increased and oxidative DNA damage, both in leukocytes and in prostate tissue, was significantly lower. Furthermore, serum levels of prostate-specific antigen (PSA) decreased after the intervention. In the other study, Kucuk et al.(15) reported that supplementation with tomato extract in men with prostate cancer modulated the grade and volume of prostate intraepithelial neoplasia and tumor, the level of serum PSA, and the level of biomarkers of cell growth and differentiation.

High lycopene intake has also been associated with lower risk for many other cancers including gastric cancer and breast cancer(16–18). In an integrated series of studies in Italy (19), tomato consumption showed a consistent inverse relationship to the risk of digestive tract tumors.

III. PHASE I AND PHASE II ENZYMES IN THE METABOLISM OF ENVIRONMENTAL CARCINOGENS

Practically all dietary and environmental carcinogens are subjected to metabolism once they enter the human body. This enzymatic process occurs mainly through oxidation as well as, to a lesser extent, reduction and hydrolysis, which transforms the chemical molecules to become more hydrophilic. This physiological event is called phase I metabolism, and is primarily catalyzed by the cytochrome P450 enzymes (CYPs). As a consequence of this enzymatic activity, procarcinogens are usually converted into highly reactive intermediates that can bind to critical macromolecules such as DNA, RNA and protein. A second group of enzymes known as phase II enzymes, conjugate reactive intermediates with endogenous cofactors, resulting in the generation of more water-soluble products which can easily be excreted in the bile or urine. The ultimate chemopreventive effects of lycopene and other carotenoids probably involve complex interactions of multiple mechanisms. However, many of their chemopreventive effects may be attributed to the enhancement of detoxification (phase II induction) as well as to the blocking of carcinogen activation (phase I inhibition) (Fig. 1).

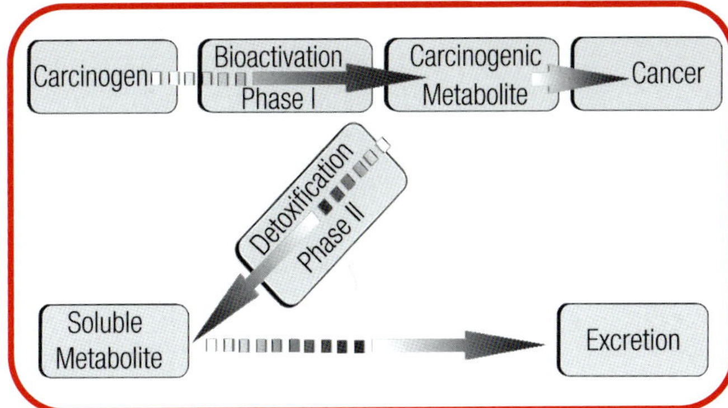

Fig. 1: The role of phase I and phase II enzymes in the metabolism of carcinogens. Carcinogens, which are usually hydrophobic compounds, are activated in the body by phase I enzymes. The activity of these enzymes leads to the formation of carcinogenic metabolites which interact with DNA to cause mutations that can lead to cancer. Induction of phase II enzymes (which conjugate reactive carcinogens to hydrophilic molecules) results in products that are readily excreted from the body.

Enhanced expression of most phase II genes such as glutathione *S*-transferase (GST), NAD[P]H: quinone reductase (NQO1), γ-glutamylcysteine synthetase (γ-GCS) and hemoxygenase-1 (HO-1) is mediated through the antioxidant responsive element (ARE). Nrf2, a member of the Cap 'n' Collar (CNC) family of leucine zipper (bZIP) transcriptional factors, dimerizes with small Maf proteins and binds to the ARE, resulting in the transcriptional activation of a battery of detoxification and antioxidant proteins (20). Nrf2 is sequestered by cytoskeleton-anchored Keap1 protein in the cytoplasm as an inactive complex. Following exposure to extracellular stimuli, Nrf2 is dissociated from Keap1 protein, translocates into the nucleus and binds to the ARE.

IV. CAROTENOIDS AND CANCER PREVENTION: INHIBITION OF TUMOR INITIATION

Some carotenoids are capable of inducing CYP enzymes, (21). While Canthaxanthin, astaxanthin and β-apo-8′-carotenal induced liver CYP1A1 and CYP1A2 in rats β-carotene, lutein and lycopene did not (22-25). In mouse liver, canthaxanthin induced weak effects whereas the other carotenoids did not stimulate CYP1A1 activity at all (26). The mechanism underlying CYP enzyme induction by carotenoids is not fully understood.

The direct effect of carotenoids on a pregnane X receptor (PXR) system, which is known to induce CYP enzymes, was tested in an *in vitro* transcription system (27). It was found that in transiently transfected HepG2 hepatoma cells, β-carotene and retinol, but not lycopene, transactivated the PXR reporter gene similarly to the positive control rifampicin. Furthermore, β-carotene caused up-regulation of CYP3A4 and CYP3A5 in these cells, pointing to a potential effect of the carotenoid on the metabolism of xenobiotics. Marked reactive oxygen species over-generation associated with CYP induction (up to 33-fold increase in the liver) was found in rats supplemented with high doses of β-carotene (28). These findings are consistent with the concept that β-carotene is potentially co-carcinogenic, and may help explain why, in large quantities, it can have harmful effects in humans as illustrated below.

It is interesting that supplementation of β-carotene to ferrets enhanced *in vitro* all-trans-retinoic acid catabolism via induction of CYPs (29) thereby reducing the protective activity of retinoic acid. These results can explain why in the well-known ATBC (30, 31) and CARET studies (32) tobacco smokers with β-carotene supplementation showed higher incidence of lung cancer. In contrast to these findings with β-carotene, moderate and high dose supplementations with lycopene substantially inhibited smoke-induced squamous metaplasia (33). This result collaborates the finding that lycopene did not affect PXR-mediated increase of CYP3A expression nor did it increase the risk for tobacco smoke induced squamous metaplasia (33).

The possible regulation of phase II enzymes by carotenoids in general and by lycopene in particular has been debated in the literature. Gradelet et al (24). have shown that canthaxanthin and astaxanthin, but not lutein and lycopene, are active in the induction of these enzymes in rats. In contrast, Bhuvaneswari et al. (34) associated the chemopreventive effect of lycopene on the incidence of DMBA-induced hamster buccal pouch tumors with a concomitant rise in the level of reduced glutathione (GSH), enzymes of the glutathione redox cycle and glutathione S-transferase in the buccal pouch mucosa. A more broad review of this subject can be found in (35).

We examined the ARE activation and its role in the induction of phase II enzymes by different tomato carotenoids (lycopene, phytoene, phytofluene and β-carotene) (36). In transiently transfected cancer cells lycopene transactivated the expression of reporter genes fused with ARE sequences. Other carotenoids such as phytoene, phytofluene, β-carotene and astaxanthin had a much lesser effect. An increase in protein as well as mRNA levels of the phase II enzymes NAD(P)H:quinone oxidoreductase (NQO1) and glutamylcysteine synthetase (GCS) was observed in non-transfected cells after carotenoid treatment. Ethanolic extract of lycopene containing unidentified hydrophilic derivatives of the carotenoid activated ARE with a similar potency to lycopene. The potency of carotenoids in ARE activation did not correlate with their effect on intracellular reactive oxygen species (ROS) and GSH level, which may indicate that ARE activation is not solely related to its antioxidant activity. Nrf2, which is found predominantly in the cytoplasm of untreated cells, translocated to the nucleus after carotenoid treatment. The increase in phase II enzymes was abolished by a dominant negative Nrf2, suggesting that carotenoid induction of these proteins depends on a functional Nrf2.

V. CAROTENOIDS AND CANCER PREVENTION: INHIBITION OF TUMOR PROMOTION AND PROGRESSION

Tumor promotion is a lengthy process in which actively proliferating preneoplastic cells accumulate and turn into a clinically apparent tumor. In some types of cancer this process may take 20-30 years. It is thus clear that reduction of cancer cell proliferation is a logical strategy to delay the onset of the disease and if the delay is long enough, even to completely prevent the development of tumors. Previous studies have suggested three possible means by which carotenoids can inhibit tumor promotion and progression: 1) restoration of gap junction communication; 2) slowdown of cell cycle progression; and 3) inhibition of the activity of hormones and growth factors which are known to promote cancer cell growth.

A. Gap junction communication

Special structures in the cell membrane, termed gap junctions, function as communication channels between cells. Normal cells are both contact-inhibited and have functional gap junctions whereas most tumor cells exhibit a reduced number of these channels. Lycopene and other carotenoids were found to induce the formation of the protein connexin 43, one of the major building blocks of these channels, thereby restoring gap junction communication (37). Downregulation of connexin 43 expression occurs early during the process of carcinogenesis. Thus lycopene and other carotenoids serve as cancer chemopreventive agents by upregulating connexin 43 expression (37). Conversely, diverse tumor promoters which stimulate cell proliferation inhibit gap junction communication (38). Based on this result, it has been hypothesized that one function of gap junction communication is to transmit growth-regulatory signals. Therefore we can conjecture that upregulation of gap junction communication is part of the mechanism by which retinoids and carotenoids may inhibit cell proliferation and reverse transformation (39). Consistent with this model of growth control, restoration of gap junction communication has been shown to result in growth arrest of neoplastic cells. Moreover, forced expression of several connexin family members in various tumor lines can restore some aspects of the normal cell phenotype [reviewed in (40)].

B. Slowdown of cell cycle progression

Lycopene has been found to inhibit proliferation of several types of cancer cells, including those of breast, prostate, lung, and endometrium. The inhibitory effects of lycopene on mammary and prostate cancer cell growth were not accompanied by apoptotic (programmed) or necrotic cell death which commonly results in response to drugs but not to dietary micronutrients. However, the inhibitory effects of lycopene on mammary and prostate cancer cell growth was accompanied by inhibition of cell cycle progression from the G0/G1 to the S phase as measured by flow cytometry (41). The inhibition of cell proliferation correlated with a decrease in cyclin D1 protein levels which is a key regulator of this process. It is well documented that growth factors affect the cell cycle apparatus primarily during G1 phase and that the main components acting as growth factor sensors are the D-type cyclins (42). Moreover, cyclin D1 is known to act as an oncogene (a gene whose dysregulation causes normal cells to become cancerous) and is found to be over-expressed in many breast cancer cell lines as well as in primary tumors (43). Thus, the decrease in cellular cyclin D1 level brought about by lycopene provides a mechanistic explanation for the anticancer activity of the carotenoid.

C. Attenuation of the cancer promoting effects of growth factors and hormones

The identification of risk factors for various types of cancer can lead to appropriate preventive measures. For example, the involvement of the sex steroids, estradiol and testosterone, for the development and progression of the specific male and female malignancies is well known. Estrogens are the most important risk factors in breast and endometrial cancer. Similarly, androgens are known to influence the development of prostate cancer. A similar role has been proposed for insulin-like growth factor-I (IGF-I) in these and in other types of cancer (see below). Thus, attenuation of the effects of these hormones and growth factors may be a central mechanism for cancer prevention by tomato lycopene.

Growth factors, either in the blood or as part of autocrine or paracrine loops, can promote cancer cell growth. Recently, it was reported that high blood levels of IGF-I existing years before malignancy detection can predict an increase in risk for breast, prostate, colorectal and lung cancer (44-47). There are two possible mechanisms that can account for the lowering of cancer risk by lycopene – to decrease IGF-I blood level, thereby diminishing the risk associated with its elevation, or to interfere with IGF-I activity in the cancer cell. In support of the first mechanism Mucci et al. reported that consumption of cooked tomatoes is substantially and significantly inversely associated with IGF-I levels (48). In addition recently, Wertz et al. supported these results by demonstrating that IGF-I expression in the rat prostate tumors was decreased by lycopene supplementation (49). Our recent results suggest that supplementation with tomato lycopene extract lowers IGF-I blood levels in colon cancer patients (unpublished results). Regarding the second mechanism, we have shown that lycopene inhibits the mitogenic action of IGF-I in human mammary cancer cells. Treatment with the carotenoid markedly reduced the intracellular signaling mechanism of IGF-I. Both tyrosine phosphorylation of insulin receptor substrate-1 and DNA binding capacity of the AP-1 transcription factor (50), downstream events in IGF-I signaling, were inhibited by lycopene.

Several epidemiological studies have searched for an association between tomato products or lycopene consumption and components of the IGF system (51, 52). While only one study found a possible association between lycopene intake and IGFBP-3 (53), other studies found that in disease-free men tomato consumption was inversely associated with IGF-I levels and/or its molar ratio with IGFBP-3 (48, 54).

Sex hormones have been demonstrated to be the most important risk factors in breast and prostate cancer. In order to establish a mechanistic link to explain the association between high lycopene consumption and reduced prostate cancer risk Wertz et al. investigated the effect of lycopene in a rat prostate tumor model (49). They found that lycopene supplementation increased necrosis rates in the prostate tumors, and that this effect was associated with a down-regulation of local androgen signaling, as well as IGF-I and IL-6 expression. The same group reported that supplementation with lycopene in young normal rats (55, 56) mildly but significantly reduced gene expression of androgen metabolizing enzymes with a reduction of active androgen also in non-cancerous prostate. These results suggest that lycopene is important for primary prostate cancer prevention. Our recent studies showed that lycopene directly inhibits androgen-induced transcriptional activity in prostate cancer cells (unpublished results). All of these mechanisms may contribute to the epidemiologically observed prostate cancer risk reduction by lycopene.

Lycopene may inhibit also estrogen-induced transcriptional activity in female hormone dependent cancers. We have already shown that various carotenoids inhibit proliferation of hormone-dependent mammary (MCF-7) and endometrial (ECC-1) cancer cells (57). Since estrogens are the most important risk factors for these malignancies, we investigated whether carotenoids attenuate estrogen induced transcriptional activity in mammary and endometrial cancer cells. Indeed, our preliminary results demonstrated that several tomato carotenoids such as lycopene, phytoene and phytofluene inhibit estrogen signaling which may explain the epidemiological observation that carotenoids reduce breast cancer risk (unpublished results).

VI. LYCOPENE BENEFITS FROM A SYNERGISTIC RELATIONSHIP WITH OTHER MICRONUTRIENTS

When reviewing data related to the chemoprevention of various diseases, it becomes evident that the use of a single carotenoid, or any other micronutrient which has been successful in *in vitro* and animal models, does not prove as favorable in human intervention studies. That is, there is no magic bullet as a cancer preventing agent, rather accumulating evidence suggests that a concerted, synergistic action of various micronutrients is more likely to be the basis of the disease-prevention activity of a diet rich in vegetables and fruit. Indeed, the sources of lycopene used in most of the human studies reviewed here were a combination of either prepared tomato products or tomato extracts containing lycopene and other tomato micronutrients and carotenoids in various proportions. For example, an oleoresin preparation used in many of these studies also contained other tomato carotenoids such as phytoene, phytofluene, and beta-carotene (Fig. 2). Pure lycopene, either from a natural or synthetic source, has rarely tested as a single agent in human prevention studies.

Fig 2: Structures of the main tomato carotenoids and their relative content in tomato lipid extract (tomato oleoresin).

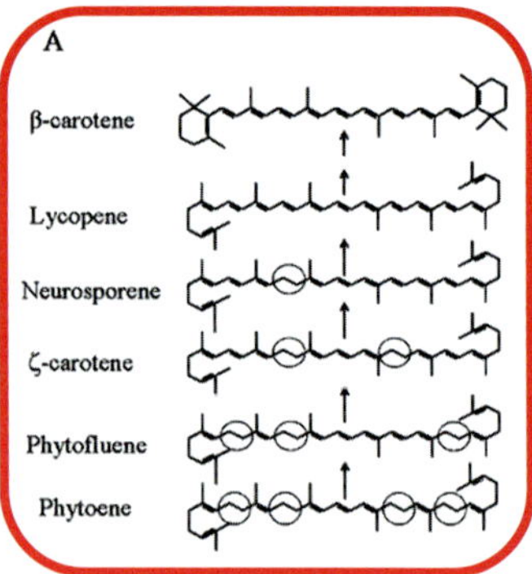

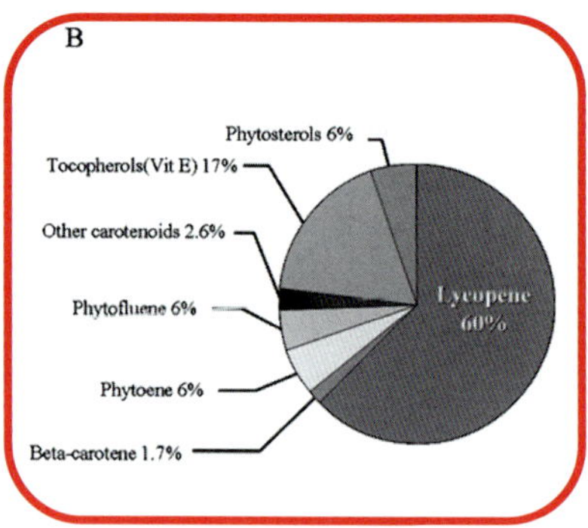

A. The structure of the main tomato carotenoids is shown together with steps in their biosynthesis. Circles depict the single bonds which are desaturated to double bonds during the synthetic pathway from phytoene to lycopene. B. The relative content of the main phytonutrients found in a tomato lipid extract. The sum of the listed compounds represent 10% of the tomato oleoresin, the rest is mainly triacyl glycerols (about 75%) and phospholipids (about 15%) (Data for the Lyc-O-Mato® preparation was provided by LycoRed, Natural Products Industries Ltd, Beer-Sheva, Israel).

The value of a concerted, synergistic action of a combination of various carotenoids and other micronutrients, was tested in skin protection from sun exposure. Sun protection activity is believed to be related to the antioxidant properties of the carotenoids. Upon UV-irradiation, the skin is exposed to photooxidative damage which is induced by the formation of reactive oxygen species. Photooxidative damage affects cellular lipids, proteins and DNA, and is considered to be involved in the pathobiochemistry of erythema formation, premature aging of the skin, development of photodermatoses, and skin cancer (58). In these experiments erythema was induced by illumination with a solar simulator, and the protective effects were investigated with β-carotene supplementation and in combination with vitamin E (59, 60). The results of these experiments show that erythema formation was significantly diminished. Moreover, erythema suppression was more pronounced with the combination of carotenoids and vitamin E.

Several studies in humans have shown that carotenoid levels in plasma and skin decrease upon UV-irradiation. Interestingly, lycopene is lost preferentially as compared to other carotenoids (61). Based on these findings which suggest that lycopene has a special role in skin protection, the beneficial, photoprotective effect of lycopene was tested. In these human experiments, three lycopene preparations were compared: lycopene alone (synthetic form), lycopene in combination with other carotenoids (tomato extract) and a third preparation containing tomato extract enriched with phytoene and phytofluene (tomato drink) (62). These three different sources containing similar amounts of lycopene (about 10 mg/day) were supplemented and after 12 weeks, significant increases in lycopene serum levels and total skin carotenoids were observed in all groups. The protective effect was significantly more pronounced in the groups that ingested the tomato extract or the drink. The difference in the efficacy of the tomato products compared to synthetic lycopene might be due to the presence of phytofluene and phytoene in the former. These results suggest that a synergistic effect of lycopene, phytofluene, and phytoene might be operative in sun skin protection.

The synergy concept was tested in a recent study (63) by comparing the potency of freeze-dried whole tomatoes (tomato powder) or pure lycopene in a rat model of prostate cancer. Rats were treated with the carcinogen NMU (N-methyl-N-nitrosourea) combined with androgens to stimulate prostate carcinogenesis, and the ability of these two preparations containing lycopene to enhance survival was compared. Mortality with prostate cancer was lower by 25% ($P = 0.09$) for rats fed the tomato powder diet than for rats fed control feed. Prostate cancer mortality of rats fed pure lycopene was similar to that of the control group. The authors concluded that consumption of tomato powder but not pure lycopene inhibited prostate carcinogenesis, suggesting that tomato products contain other compounds besides lycopene, that modify prostate carcinogenesis. In an accompanying editorial, Gann et al.(64) pointed out that carotenoids and other secondary plant compounds have evolved as sets of interacting compounds, a complexity that limits the usefulness of reductionist approaches seeking to identify single protective compounds.

VII. CONCLUDING REMARKS

Although cancer prevention by dietary means is today widely accepted (5 a day), an overwhelming need still exists to search for more effective dietary preventive agents and to use them in synergistic combinations. Development of 'combination prevention' will be just as essential for cancer prevention as combination chemotherapy has been in the treatment of malignant diseases. The effective blend of nutrients, composed in the tomato by 'mother nature', is an important example of the combination prevention concept.

REFERENCES:

1. Sporn, M. B. and Newton, D. L. Chemoprevention of cancer with retinoids, Fed Proc. *38:* 2528-34, 1979.
2. Moolgavkar, S. H. The multistage theory of carcinogenesis and the age distribution of cancer in man, J Natl Cancer Inst. *61:* 49-52, 1978.
3. Surh, Y. J. Cancer chemoprevention with dietary phytochemicals, Nat Rev Cancer. *3:* 768-80, 2003.
4. Wattenberg, L. W., Hanley, A. B., Barany, G., Sparnins, V. L., Lam, L. K., and Fenwick, G. R. Inhibition of carcinogenesis by some minor dietary constituents, Princess Takamatsu Symp. *16:* 193-203, 1985.
5. Manson, M. M., Gescher, A., Hudson, E. A., Plummer, S. M., Squires, M. S., andPrigent, S. A. Blocking and suppressing mechanisms of chemoprevention by dietary constituents, Toxicol Lett. *112-113:* 499-505, 2000.
6. Lee, J. M. and Johnson, J. A. An important role of Nrf2-ARE pathway in the cellular defense mechanism, J Biochem Mol Biol. *37:* 139-43, 2004.
7. Lee, J. S. and Surh, Y. J. Nrf2 as a novel molecular target for chemoprevention, Cancer Lett. *224:* 171-84, 2005.
8. Chen, C. and Kong, A. N. Dietary chemopreventive compounds and ARE/EpRE signaling, Free Radic Biol Med. *36:* 1505-16, 2004.
9. Bertram, J. S. Carotenoids and gene regulation, Nutr Rev. *57:* 182-91, 1999.
10. Kelloff, G. J., Sigman, C. C., and Greenwald, P. Cancer chemoprevention: progress and promise, Eur J Cancer. *35:* 1755-62, 1999.
11. Sporn, M. B. and Suh, N. Chemoprevention: an essential approach to controlling cancer, Nat Rev Cancer. *2:* 537-43, 2002.
12. Giovannucci, E. Tomatoes, tomato-based products, lycopene, and cancer: review of the epidemiologic literature, J Natl Cancer Inst. *91:* 317-331, 1999.
13. Grant, W. B. An ecologic study of dietary links to prostate cancer, Altern Med Rev. *4:* 162-9, 1999.
14. Chen, L., Stacewicz-Sapuntzakis, M., Duncan, C., Sharifi, R., Ghosh, L., van Breemen, R., Ashton, D., and Bowen, P. E. Oxidative DNA damage in prostate cancer patients consuming tomato sauce- based entrees as a whole-food intervention, J Natl Cancer Inst. *93:* 1872-9., 2001.
15. Kucuk, O., Sarkar, F. H., Sakr, W., et al. Phase II randomized clinical trial of lycopene supplementation before radical prostatectomy, Cancer Epidemiol Biomarkers Prev. *10:* 861-8., 2001.
16. Tsubono, Y., Tsugane, S., and Gey, K. F. Plasma antioxidant vitamins and carotenoids in five Japanese populations with varied mortality from gastric cancer, Nutr Cancer. *34:* 56-61, 1999.
17. Ronco, A., De Stefani, E., Boffetta, P., Deneo-Pellegrini, H., Mendilaharsu, M., and Leborgne, F. Vegetables, fruits, and related nutrients and risk of breast cancer: a case-control study in Uruguay, Nutr Cancer. *35:* 111-9, 1999.
18. Hulten, K., Van Kappel, A. L., Winkvist, A., Kaaks, R., Hallmans, G., Lenner, P., and Riboli, E. Carotenoids, alpha-tocopherols, and retinol in plasma and breast cancer risk in northern Sweden, Cancer Causes Control. *12:* 529-37, 2001.
19. La Vecchia, C. Tomatoes, lycopene intake, and digestive tract and female hormone-related neoplasms, Exp Biol Med (Maywood). *227:* 860-3, 2002.

20. Keum, Y. S., Jeong, W. S., and Kong, A. N. Chemoprevention by isothiocyanates and their underlying molecular signaling mechanisms, Mutat Res. *555:* 191-202, 2004.
21. Sharoni, Y., Danilenko, M., Dubi, N., Ben-Dor, A., and Levy, J. Carotenoids and transcription, Arch Biochem Biophys. *430:* 89-96, 2004.
22. Astorg, P., Berges, R., and Suschetet, M. Induction of gamma GT- and GST-P positive foci in the liver of rats treated with 2-nitropropane or propane 2-nitronate, Cancer Lett. *79:* 101-6, 1994.
23. Astorg, P., Gradelet, S., Leclerc, J., Canivenc, M. C., and Siess, M. H. Effects of beta-carotene and canthaxanthin on liver xenobiotic-metabolizing enzymes in the rat, Food Chem Toxicol. *32:* 735-42, 1994.
24. Gradelet, S., Leclerc, J., Siess, M. H., and Astorg, P. O. beta-Apo-8'-carotenal, but not beta-carotene, is a strong inducer of liver cytochromes P4501A1 and 1A2 in rat, Xenobiotica. *26:* 909-19, 1996.
25. Gradelet, S., Astorg, P., Leclerc, J., Chevalier, J., Vernevaut, M. F., and Siess, M. H. Effects of canthaxanthin, astaxanthin, lycopene and lutein on liver xenobiotic-metabolizing enzymes in the rat, Xenobiotica. *26:* 49-63, 1996.
26. Astorg, P., Gradelet, S., Leclerc, J., and Siess, M. H. Effects of provitamin A or non-provitamin A carotenoids on liver xenobiotic-metabolizing enzymes in mice, Nutr Cancer. *27:* 245-9, 1997.
27. Ruhl, R., Sczech, R., Landes, N., Pfluger, P., Kluth, D., and Schweigert, F. J. Carotenoids and their metabolites are naturally occurring activators of gene expression via the pregnane X receptor, Eur J Nutr. *43:* 336-43, 2004.
28. Paolini, M., Antelli, A., Pozzetti, L., Spetlova, D., Perocco, P., Valgimigli, L., Pedulli, G. F., and Cantelli-Forti, G. Induction of cytochrome P450 enzymes and over-generation of oxygen radicals in beta-carotene supplemented rats, Carcinogenesis. *22:* 1483-95, 2001.
29. Liu, C., Russell, R. M., and Wang, X. D. Exposing ferrets to cigarette smoke and a pharmacological dose of beta-carotene supplementation enhance in vitro retinoic acid catabolism in lungs via induction of cytochrome P450 enzymes, J Nutr. *133:* 173-9, 2003.
30. Albanes, D., Heinonen, O. P., Taylor, P. R., et al. Alpha-Tocopherol and beta-carotene supplements and lung cancer incidence in the alpha-tocopherol, beta-carotene cancer prevention study: effects of base-line characteristics and study compliance, J Natl Cancer Inst. *88:* 1560-70, 1996.
31. Albanes, D., Heinonen, O. P., Huttunen, J. K., et al. Effects of alpha-tocopherol and beta-carotene supplements on cancer incidence in the Alpha-Tocopherol Beta-Carotene Cancer Prevention Study, Am J Clin Nutr. *62:* 1427S-1430S, 1995.
32. Omenn, G. S., Goodman, G. E., Thornquist, M. D., et al. Effects of a combination of beta carotene and vitamin A on lung cancer and cardiovascular disease, New Engl J Med. *334:* 1150-5, 1996.
33. Liu, C., Lian, F., Smith, D. E., Russell, R. M., and Wang, X. D. Lycopene supplementation inhibits lung squamous metaplasia and induces apoptosis via up-regulating insulin-like growth factor-binding protein 3 in cigarette smoke-exposed ferrets, Cancer Res. *63:* 3138-44, 2003.
34. Bhuvaneswari, V., Velmurugan, B., Balasenthil, S., Ramachandran, C. R., and Nagini, S. Chemopreventive efficacy of lycopene on 7,12-dimethylbenz[a]anthracene-induced hamster buccal pouch carcinogenesis, Fitoterapia. *72:* 865-74, 2001.

35. Sharoni, Y., Agbaria, R., Amir, H., et al. Regulation of transcription by antioxidant carotenoids. *In:* L. Packer, U. Obermueller-Jevic, K. Kraemer, and H. Sies (eds.), Carotenoids and Retinoids: Biological Actions and Human Health, pp. 261-274. Champaign, IL: AOCS press, 2004.
36. Ben-Dor, A., Steiner, M., Gheber, L., Danilenko, M., Dubi, N., Linnewiel, K., Zick, A., Sharoni, Y., and Levy, J. Carotenoids activate the antioxidant response element transcription system, Mol Cancer Ther. *4:* 177-86, 2005.
37. Zhang, L. X., Cooney, R. V., and Bertram, J. S. Carotenoids up-regulate connexin-43 gene expression independent of their provitamin-A or antioxidant properties, Cancer Res. *52:* 5707-5712, 1992.
38. Matesic, D. F., Rupp, H. L., Bonney, W. J., Ruch, R. J., and Trosko, J. E. Changes in gap-junction permeability, phosphorylation, and number mediated by phorbol ester and non-phorbol-ester tumor promoters in rat liver epithelial cells, Mol Carcinog. *10:* 226-36, 1994.
39. Vine, A. L. and Bertram, J. S. Upregulation of Connexin 43 by Retinoids but Not by Non-Provitamin A Carotenoids Requires RARs, Nutr Cancer. *52:* 105-13, 2005.
40. Vine, A. L. and Bertram, J. S. Cancer chemoprevention by connexins, Cancer Metastasis Rev. *21:* 199-216, 2002.
41. Nahum, A., Hirsch, K., Danilenko, M., Watts, C. K., Prall, O. W., Levy, J., and Sharoni, Y. Lycopene inhibition of cell cycle progression in breast and endometrial cancer cells is associated with reduction in cyclin D levels and retention of p27(Kip1) in the cyclin E-cdk2 complexes, Oncogene. *20:* 3428-36., 2001.
42. Sherr, C. J. D-type cyclins, Trends Biochem Sci. *20:* 187-190, 1995.
43. Buckley, M. F., Sweeney, K. J., Hamilton, J. A., et al. Expression and amplification of cyclin genes in human breast cancer, Oncogene. *8:* 2127-2133, 1993.
44. Mantzoros, C. S., Tzonou, A., Signorello, L. B., Stampfer, M., Trichopoulos, D., and Adami, H. O. Insulin-like growth factor 1 in relation to prostate cancer and benign prostatic hyperplasia, Br J Cancer. *76:* 1115-8, 1997.
45. Hankinson, S. E., Willett, W. C., Colditz, G. A., Hunter, D. J., Michaud, D. S., Deroo, B., Rosner, B., Speizer, F. E., and Pollak, M. Circulating concentrations of insulin-like growth factor I and risk of breast cancer, Lancet. *351:* 1393-1396, 1998.
46. Ma, J., Pollak, M. N., Giovannucci, E., Chan, J. M., Tao, Y., Hennekens, C. H., and Stampfer, M. J. Prospective study of colorectal cancer risk in men and plasma levels of insulin-like growth factor (IGF)-I and IGF-binding protein-3, J Natl Cancer Inst. *91:* 620-5, 1999.
47. Yu, H., Spitz, M. R., Mistry, J., Gu, J., Hong, W. K., and Wu, X. Plasma levels of insulin-like growth factor-I and lung cancer risk: a case-control analysis, J Natl Cancer Inst. *91:* 151-156, 1999.
48. Mucci, L. A., Tamimi, R., Lagiou, P., Trichopoulou, A., Benetou, V., Spanos, E., and Trichopoulos, D. Are dietary influences on the risk of prostate cancer mediated through the insulin-like growth factor system? BJU Int. *87:* 814-20., 2001.
49. Siler, U., Barella, L., Spitzer, V., Schnorr, J., Lein, M., Goralczyk, R., and Wertz, K. Lycopene and Vitamin E interfere with autocrine/paracrine loops in the Dunning prostate cancer model, Faseb J 1019-21, 2004.
50. Karas, M., Amir, H., Fishman, D., et al. Lycopene interferes with cell cycle progression and insulin-like growth factor I signaling in mammary cancer cells, Nutr Cancer. *36:* 101-111, 2000.

51. Signorello, L. B., Kuper, H., Lagiou, P., Wuu, J., Mucci, L. A., Trichopoulos, D., and Adami, H. O. Lifestyle factors and insulin-like growth factor 1 levels among elderly men, Eur J Cancer Prev. *9:* 173-8, 2000.
52. Vrieling, A., Voskuil, D. W., Bueno de Mesquita, H. B., Kaaks, R., van Noord, P. A., Keinan-Boker, L., van Gils, C. H., and Peeters, P. H. Dietary determinants of circulating insulin-like growth factor (IGF)-I and IGF binding proteins 1, -2 and -3 in women in the Netherlands, Cancer Causes Control. *15:* 787-96, 2004.
53. Holmes, M. D., Pollak, M. N., Willett, W. C., and Hankinson, S. E. Dietary correlates of plasma insulin-like growth factor I and insulin-like growth factor binding protein 3 concentrations, Cancer Epidemiol Biomarkers Prev. *11:* 852-61, 2002.
54. Gunnell, D., Oliver, S. E., Peters, T. J., et al. Are diet-prostate cancer associations mediated by the IGF axis? A cross-sectional analysis of diet, IGF-I and IGFBP-3 in healthy middle-aged men, Br J Cancer. *88:* 1682-6, 2003.
55. Herzog, A., Siler, U., Spitzer, V., Seifert, N., Denelavas, A., Buchwald Hunziker, P., Hunziker, W., Goralczyk, R., and Wertz, K. Lycopene reduced gene expression of steroid targets and inflammatory markers in normal rat prostate, Faseb J, 2004.
56. Wertz, K., Siler, U., and Goralczyk, R. Lycopene: modes of action to promote prostate health, Arch Biochem Biophys. *430:* 127-34, 2004.
57. Levy, J., Bosin, E., Feldman, B., Giat, Y., Miinster, A., Danilenko, M., and Sharoni, Y. Lycopene is a more potent inhibitor of human cancer cell proliferation than either α-carotene or β-carotene., Nutr Cancer. *24:* 257-267, 1995.
58. Berneburg, M. and Krutmann, J. Photoimmunology, DNA repair and photocarcinogenesis, J Photochem Photobiol B. *54:* 87-93, 2000.
59. Stahl, W., Heinrich, U., Jungmann, H., Sies, H., and Tronnier, H. Carotenoids and carotenoids plus vitamin E protect against ultraviolet light-induced erythema in humans, Am J Clin Nutr. *71:* 795-8, 2000.
60. Sies, H. and Stahl, W. Nutritional protection against skin damage from sunlight, Annu Rev Nutr. *24:* 173-200, 2004.
61. Ribaya Mercado, J. D., Garmyn, M., Gilchrest, B. A., and Russell, R. M. Skin lycopene is destroyed preferentially over beta-carotene during ultraviolet irradiation in humans, J Nutr.*125*:1854-9,1995.
62. Aust, O., Stahl, W., Sies, H., Tronnier, H., and Heinrich, U. Supplementation with tomato-based products increases lycopene, phytofluene, and phytoene levels in human serum and protects against UV-light-induced erythema, Int J Vitam Nutr Res. 75: 54-60, 2005.
63. Boileau, T. W., Liao, Z., Kim, S., Lemeshow, S., Erdman, J. W., Jr., and Clinton, S. K. Prostate carcinogenesis in N-methyl-N-nitrosourea (NMU)-testosterone-treated rats fed tomato powder, lycopene, or energy-restricted diets, J Natl Cancer Inst. 95: 1578-86, 2003.
64. Gann, P. H. and Khachik, F. Tomatoes or lycopene versus prostate cancer: is evolution anti-reductionist? J Natl Cancer Inst. 95: 1563-5, 2003.

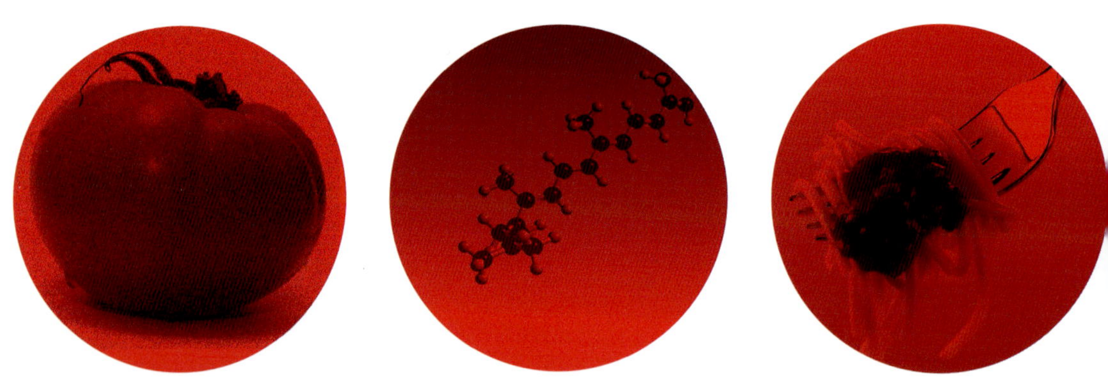

The Role of Tomato Lycopene in the Treatment of Prostate Cancer

Dr. Elisabeth Heath[1]
Dr. Soley Seren[1]
Dr. Kazim Sahin[2]
Dr. Omer Kucuk[1]
[1]Division of Hematology and Oncology, Department of Medicine
Wayne State University and Barbara Ann Karmanos Cancer Institute, Detroit, Michigan,United States
[2]Department of Animal Nutrition, Faculty of Veterinary Science, Firat University, Elazig, Turkey

Abstract

Dietary intake of lycopene is inversely associated with the risk of prostate cancer. Preclinical studies show that lycopene has potent *in vitro* and *in vivo* anti-tumor effects on prostate cancer cells suggesting potential preventive and therapeutic roles for lycopene. However, small number and size of clinical trials conducted with lycopene preclude firm conclusions with regard to its use in prostate cancer prevention and treatment in humans. Further research, including hypothesis driven mechanistic studies as well as larger randomized clinical intervention trials with lycopene in prostate cancer are warranted.

INTRODUCTION

Prostate cancer is the second leading cause of cancer deaths in males in the United States. It accounts for about thirty percent of all cancers that are diagnosed in men. In 2001, the American Cancer Society has predicted 198,100 new cases and 31,500 deaths from prostate cancer in the US (1). The incidence of prostate cancer has increased dramatically in the last decade due mainly to the increase in screening using prostate specific antigen. The prevalence of the precursor lesion, high grade prostatic intraepithelial neoplasia (HGPIN) and carcinoma of the prostate increase with aging starting in men in their early thirties (2). Knowledge of the natural history of development, elucidation of critical genetic and epigenetic pathways and presence of risk factors for identifying target populations make prostate cancer a good target for prevention (3). Thus, there is great interest in prostate cancer chemoprevention, which can be defined as the administration of natural and/or synthetic agents that inhibit one or more steps in prostate carcinogenesis (4).

Prostate Cancer Chemoprevention

Before embarking on large chemoprevention clinical trials intermediate endpoints or surrogate endpoint biomarkers (SEBs) could be used in small efficient phase I-II clinical chemoprevention trials to explore the efficacy and elucidate the mechanisms of action of potential chemopreventive compounds. Gap junctional intercellular communication (GJIC) and Cx expression levels could be useful intermediate endpoints in prostate cancer chemoprevention clinical trials, because they are decreased in prostate cancer cells (5-7). Therefore chemopreventive agents modulating Cx expression and/or GJIC would be of great interest (8,9). Retinoids and carotenoids are among potent upregulators of Cx43 and GJIC (10-12). In particular, lycopene increases gap junctional intercellular communication by increasing expression of gap junctional gene, connexin 43 (10,13,14). This action correlates strongly with the ability of lycopene and other carotenoids to suppress neoplastic transformation in model cell culture systems (10). This action of carotenoids has been proposed to have mechanistic significance by enabling the transfer of growth-regulatory signals between normal growth-inhibited cells and pre-neoplastic cells. Indeed, when neoplastic cells were forced into junctional communication with quiescent normal cells, the neoplastic cells became growth arrested in direct proportion to their extent of junctional communication (8). Progressive decreases with disease severity in the expression of Cx43 have been reported in the human prostate (5), and there is evidence in prostatic carcinoma cell lines that some of this loss of junctional communication may result from defects in assembly of Cx43 protein into gap junctions (6). When functional communication was restored in a human prostatic carcinoma cell line, cells had more normal differentiation, reduced proliferation and suppressed tumorigenicity (7). Therefore, Cx43 and GJIC could be used as SEBs or intermediate endpoints in phase II clinical chemoprevention trials for prostate cancer.

It would be important to identify men at high risk for prostate cancer to enroll in chemoprevention trials. In addition to presence of HGPIN in the prostate and elevated serum PSA levels, recent studies suggest high serum IGF-1 and/or low serum IGFBP-3 as good markers for high prostate cancer risk. Insulin-like growth factors have mitogenic and antiapoptotic effects on normal and transformed prostate epithelial cells (15-17). IGF-1 is an important mitogen for prostate cells. IGFBPs have opposing actions, in part by binding IGF-1, but also by direct inhibitory effects on target cells (15). In recent epidemiologic studies, relatively high plasma IGF-1 and low IGFBP-3 levels have been independently associated with greater risk of prostate cancer (18-22). Two- to four-fold elevated risk has been observed for prostate cancer in men in the top quartile of IGF-1 relative to those in the bottom quartile, and low levels of IGFBP-3 were associated with an approximate doubling of risk (18). Recent data show that lycopene administration to humans with colon cancer for 1-5 weeks prior to surgery significantly reduces serum IGF-1 levels (23).

Since prostate carcinogenesis is a multistep process and takes many years to occur in humans, it is an ideal disease to conduct clinical chemoprevention trials. Currently there are no chemopreventive agents approved by United States Food and Drug Administration for prostate cancer. Chemopreventive agents to be investigated should be non-toxic, inexpensive and available for use by mouth, because they are expected to be used by healthy people in the general population.

LYCOPENE

Epidemiological studies have shown an inverse association between dietary intake of tomatoes, tomato products, lycopene and prostate cancer (PCA) risk (24-27). Lycopene, the major carotenoid in tomatoes, has been postulated to be the protective compound against prostate cancer (24-28). Possible mechanisms of action for lycopene include (a) inhibition of growth and induction of differentiation in cancer cells by modulating the expression of cell cycle regulatory proteins (29-33), (b) modulation of the IGF-1/IGFBP-3 system (15, 18-22, 33-36), (c) up-regulation of tumor suppressor protein Cx43 and increased gap junctional intercellular communication (8-10, 13, 14, 37-44), (d) modulation of redox signalling (45), (e) prevention of oxidative DNA damage (46,47), and (f) modulation of carcinogen metabolising enzymes (48).

Lycopene is a potent antioxidant and quencher of singlet oxygen (49,50) and a predominant of various carotenoids in human prostate glands obtained by radical prostatectomy from patients with PCa (51). Lycopene and beta-carotene were the predominant carotenoids, with means $\pm$ SE of 0.80 $\pm$ 0.08 and 0.54 $\pm$ 0.09 nmol/g, respectively. The presence of lycopene in the prostate at concentrations that are biologically active in laboratory studies supports the hypothesis that lycopene may have direct effects within the prostate and contribute to the reduced prostate cancer risk associated with the consumption of tomato-based products. Intake of encapsulated lycopene can increase the serum levels of lycopene within days (52). Rao et al (52) provided 19 healthy human subjects with tomato juice, spaghetti sauce, and tomato oleoresin capsules (Lyc-O-Mato®) and observed a two-fold increase in serum lycopene level and diminished amounts of serum thiobarbituric acid-reactive substances, a biomarker of oxidative stress. The same group observed significantly lower serum and prostate tissue lycopene levels (44%, $p = 0.04$; 78%, $p = 0.05$, respectively) in patients with PCa than in their controls in a case-control study (53).

Clinical trials with lycopene

Despite the inverse association between lycopene intake and prostate cancer observed in epidemiological studies, few clinical intervention studies have reported the effects of lycopene supplements in men with prostate cancer. Kucuk et al (54) conducted a randomized clinical trial to investigate the effect of lycopene supplementation on the cancerous and benign prostate tissues and on serum levels of PSA, IGF-1 and IGFBP-3 of patients with prostate cancer. They hypothesized that lycopene supplementation would decrease growth and induce apoptosis in premalignant and malignant prostate cells by up-regulating Cx43, down-regulating IGF-1 and decreasing the ratio of bcl-2/bax in patients with localized prostate cancer. They conducted a randomized, two-arm intervention study. Patients with a diagnosis of prostate cancer who were scheduled to undergo radical prostatectomy were randomly assigned to either lycopene supplementation or no intervention for three weeks prior to surgery. At baseline, patients gave a blood sample and completed a food frequency questionnaire. Another blood sample was obtained for biomarker studies after three weeks immediately before surgery. Then the patients had radical prostatectomy and the prostate specimens were step-sectioned, entirely embedded and evaluated for pathologic stage, Gleason score, the volume of prostate cancer as well as the extent of HGPIN in the gland. The specimens were examined for biomarkers of cell differentiation and apoptosis. Comparisons were made between intervention and control groups. Biomarkers of differentiation (Cx43) and apoptosis (bcl-2 and bax) were assessed by Western blotting in benign and malignant tissue samples obtained from radical prostatectomy specimens. Plasma lycopene levels were measured at baseline and after three weeks of intervention and tissue lycopene levels were measured in benign tissue samples obtained from prostatectomy specimens. Subjects randomized to the intervention arm were given a supply of 15 mg lycopene capsules (Lyc-O-Mato®, LycoRed Natural Products Industries, Beer-Sheva, Israel). Subjects randomized to the control arm were asked to continue their regular diet and were given the NCI recommendations to increase daily fruit and vegetable intake to 5 servings a day. Subjects randomized to the intervention arm were asked to take one lycopene capsule twice daily with meals.

Although the study goal was to investigate the modulation of biomarkers, Kucuk et al (54) found remarkable changes in clinical endpoints. They found that the plasma PSA level decreased by 18% in the intervention group, while it increased by 14% in the control group over the study period ($p = 0.22$). In the intervention group, 11 of 15 patients (73%) had involvement of surgical margins and/or extra-prostatic tissues with cancer, compared to 2 of 11 patients (18%) in the control group ($p = 0.02$). 12 of 15 patients (80%) in the lycopene group had tumors that measured 4 cc or less, compared to 5 of 11 (45%) in the control group ($p = 0.22$). Multifocal and/or diffuse involvement by HGPIN was observed in 10 of 15 subjects (67%) in the lycopene group, compared to all 11 subjects (100%) in the control group ($p = 0.05$).

There were also interesting changes in the biomarkers in the lycopene arm. The expression of gap junctional protein, Cx43, in the malignant part of the prostate glands, was 0.63 ± 0.19 OD units in the lycopene group compared to the 0.25 ± 0.08 OD units in the control group ($p=0.13$). The expression of two important cell cycle regulatory proteins, bcl-2 and bax, were not significantly different between the two groups, although the level of bax appeared to be higher in the lycopene group (1.05 ± 0.29) compared to the control group (0.68 ± 0.18). The expression of Cx43 was 0.64 ± 0.12 in the lycopene group compared to 0.51 ± 0.10 in the control group. The expression of bcl-2 was 0.63 ± 0.04 in the intervention group and 0.58 ± 0.04 in the control group ($p=0.31$), and the expression of bax was 0.62 ± 0.10 in the intervention group and 0.79 ± 0.11 in the control group ($p=0.28$). Plasma level of IGF-1 decreased by 29% (from 233 ± 21 ng/ml to 169 ± 23 ng/ml) in the lycopene group ($p=0.0002$) and by 30% (from 199 ± 20 ng/ml to 140 ± 16 ng/ml) in the control group ($p=0.0003$). Interestingly, a similar degree of reduction in IGF-1 was observed in both groups. IGFBP-3 levels also decreased in both intervention (25%) and control (21%) groups during the study period. The decreases in the plasma IGFBP-3 levels in the intervention (from 5230 ng/ml to 3924 ng/ml) and control groups (5200 ng/ml to 4070 ng/ml) were statistically significant ($p=0.0002$ and $p=0.0001$, respectively). Prostatic tissue lycopene levels were 47% higher in the intervention group (0.53 ± 0.03 ng/gm of prostate tissue) compared to control group (0.36 ± 0.06), which was a significant difference ($p = 0.02$).

The results suggest that oral intake of 15 mg of lycopene twice daily for three weeks may be sufficient to modulate clinical markers of disease. The microscopic extension of prostate cancer to surgical margins and/or to extra-prostatic tissues appeared to have decreased as a result of lycopene supplementation. Patients in the lycopene group had a decrease in the plasma PSA level, which is a parameter of prostate cancer burden. The implication of these results is that lycopene may have an antitumor effect and thus may even be useful as an adjunct to standard treatments of prostate cancer, such as surgery, radiation therapy, hormones and chemotherapy. In addition, lycopene supplementation appears to have reduced the diffuse involvement of the prostate gland with HGPIN, which is widely accepted as a precursor of prostate cancer (55). HGPIN has been proposed as an intermediate endpoint in chemoprevention studies (55). Diffuse and/or multifocal involvement of the prostate with HGPIN was less common among patients randomized to the lycopene arm compared to the control subjects on the study. This finding suggests that lycopene may prevent the development of prostate cancer by decreasing HGPIN. Furthermore, the modulation of HGPIN by lycopene supports the hypothesis that HGPIN is a suitable intermediate endpoint for prostate cancer chemoprevention trials.

Chen et al (56) conducted a similar clinical trial to examine the effects of consumption of tomato sauce-based pasta dishes on lycopene uptake, oxidative DNA damage, and prostate-specific antigen (PSA) levels in patients with prostate cancer. Thirty-two patients with localized prostate adenocarcinoma consumed tomato sauce-based pasta dishes for the 3 weeks (30 mg of lycopene per day) preceding their scheduled radical prostatectomy. Serum and prostate lycopene concentrations, serum PSA levels, and leukocyte DNA oxidative damage (ratio of 8-hydroxy-2'-deoxyguanosine [8-OHdG] to 2'-deoxyguanosine [dG]) were assessed before and after the dietary intervention. DNA oxidative damage was assessed in resected prostate tissue from study participants and from seven randomly selected prostate cancer patients. After the dietary intervention, serum and prostate lycopene concentrations were statistically significantly increased, from 638 nM to 1258 nM (P<0.001) and from 0.28 nmol/g to 0.82 nmol/g (P <0.001), respectively. Compared with preintervention levels, leukocyte oxidative DNA damage was statistically significantly reduced after the intervention, from 0.61 8-OHdG/10^5 dG to 0.48 8-OHdG/ 10^5 dG (P =0.005). Furthermore, prostate tissue oxidative DNA damage was also statistically significantly lower in men who had the intervention (0.76 8-OHdG/10^5 dG than in the randomly selected patients (1.06 8-OHdG/10^5 dG (P =0.03). Serum PSA levels decreased after the intervention, from 10.9 ng/ml (95% CI = 8.7 to 13.2 ng/ml) to 8.7 ng/ml (95% CI = 6.8 to 10.6 ng/ml) (P<0.001). These data also support a possible role for a tomato sauce constituent, possibly lycopene, in the treatment of prostate cancer and warrant further testing.

Ansari and Gupta (57) compared the efficacy of lycopene plus orchiectomy with orchiectomy alone in the management of advanced prostate cancer. Fifty-four patients with metastatic prostatic cancer were entered into the trial. Patients were randomized to orchiectomy alone (n=27) or orchiectomy plus lycopene (n=27). Lycopene was started on the day of orchiectomy at 2 mg twice daily. At 6 months there was a significant reduction in PSA level in both treatments, but more marked in the lycopene group (mean 9.1 and 26.4 ng/ml, P = 0.9). After 2 years these changes were more consistent in the lycopene group (mean 3.01 and 9.02 ng/ml; P < 0.001). 11 (40%) patients in orchiectomy and 21 (78%) in the lycopene group had a complete PSA response (P < 0.05), with a partial response in 9 (33%) and 4

(15%), and progression in 7 (25%) and 2 (7%), respectively ($P < 0.05$). Bone scans showed that in the orchiectomy arm only 4 (15%) patients had a complete response, and in the lycopene group 8 (30%) had a complete response ($P < 0.02$); additionally partial responses were observed in 19 (70%) and 17 (63%) patients, and progression in 4 (15%) and 2 (7%) patients in orchiectomy and lycopene groups respectively ($P < 0.02$). There was a significant improvement in peak urine flow rate in the lycopene group ($P < 0.04$). 12 (22%) patients in orchiectomy group and 7 (13%) in lycopene group died ($P < 0.001$). The authors concluded that adding lycopene to orchiectomy produced a more consistent decrease in serum PSA level, provided better relief from bone pain and lower urinary tract symptoms, and improved survival compared with orchiectomy alone.

MECHANISMS

Evolving evidence suggests that carotenoids may modulate processes related to mutagenesis, carcinogenesis, cell differentiation, and proliferation independently of their role as antioxidants or precursors of vitamin A (8-10, 13, 14, 31, 37-44, 58-60). One action of lycopene, as well as many other carotenoids, is to increase gap junctional intercellular communication by increasing expression of a widely-expressed gap junctional gene, connexin 43 (10,13-14). This action correlates strongly with the ability of these carotenoids to suppress neoplastic transformation in model cell culture systems (14), an action which is shared by retinoids (9). This action of carotenoids has been proposed to have mechanistic significance by enabling the transfer of growth-regulatory signals between normal growth-inhibited cells and pre-neoplastic cells. Indeed, when neoplastic cells were forced into junctional communication with quiescent normal cells, the neoplastic cells became growth arrested in direct proportion to their extent of junctional communication (41). Consistent with the hypothesis of growth control via junctional communication, first proposed by Loewenstein (42), have been multiple reports that connexin expression and/or junctional communication is severely impaired in most solid tumors (reviewed in 61). Progressive decreases with disease severity in the expression of Cx43 have been reported in the human prostate (5), and there is evidence in prostatic carcinoma cell lines that some of this loss of junctional communication may result from defects in assembly of Cx43 protein into gap junctions (6). When functional communication was restored in a human prostatic carcinoma cell line, cells had more normal differentiation, reduced proliferation and suppressed tumorigenicity (7).

Insulin-like growth factors have mitogenic and antiapoptotic effects on normal and transformed prostate epithelial cells (15-17). While most circulating IGF-1 originates in the liver, IGF bioactivity in tissues is related to both circulating levels of IGF and IGFBP as well as local production of IGFs, IGFBPs, and IGFBP proteases (62). Whereas IGF-1 is an important mitogen for prostate cells, IGFBPs have opposing actions, in part by binding IGF-1, but also by direct inhibitory effects on target cells. As mitogens and anti-apoptotic agents, IGFs may be important in carcinogenesis, possibly by increasing the risk of cellular transformation by enhancing cell turnover. In recent epidemiologic studies, relatively high IGF-1 and low IGFBP-3 plasma levels have been independently associated with greater risk of prostate cancer (18-22).

A possible mechanism for the observed decrease in tumor parameters is up-regulation of Cx43 (54). Decreased expression of connexins, including Cx43 has been widely reported in human tumors in comparison to normal tissue (61), and connexins are regarded by many as putative tumor suppressor genes (63,64). Increased expression of Cx43 in tumor tissue in the intervention group, although not reaching statistical significance, perhaps because of the small number of subjects, may have mechanistic importance to the observed differences in pathology between these two groups. Increased expression of Cx43 and resulting increases in GJC have previously been shown to occur after treatment of human and murine cells in culture with diverse carotenoids, including lycopene (14). Up-regulated junctional communication has in turn been linked to decreased proliferation in normal and pre-neoplastic cells (65). Furthermore, recent studies have shown that in human carcinoma cells, genetically engineered to be inducible for Cx43 expression, gene induction leads to decreases in their neoplastic potential as measured by changes in anchorage-independent growth and by growth as tumors in the nude mouse (66). Previously, others have reported that Cx43 expression is progressively decreased in the prostate with increased disease severity, implying that Cx43 expression is negatively selected during tumor progression (5). Similar reductions have been seen in tumor vs. normal prostate cells (67). The concept of negative selection during disease progression received support from studies demonstrating that the forced expression of Cx43 in a human prostatic carcinoma cell line results in decreased neoplastic potential of these cells (7).

CONCLUSION

Lycopene supplementation may decrease the growth of prostate cancer, perhaps due to up-regulation of Cx43, decrease in IGF-1 or increase in IGFBP-3. Other potential mechanisms include modulation of oxidative stress, inflammation, PPAR-γ, RAR or RXR pathways. Small clinical trials suggest potential preventive and therapeutic effects of lycopene on prostate cancer in humans. If confirmed by larger randomized clinical trials lycopene could become a useful agent in prostate cancer prevention and/or treatment. The efficacy as well as the appropriate dose and duration of lycopene supplementation remain to be determined.

REFERENCES:

1. Greenlee RT, Hill-Harmon MB, Murray T, Thun M: Cancer statistics, 2001. CA Cancer J Clin 51:15-36, 2001
2. Sakr WA, Haas GP, Cassin BJ, Pontes JE, Crissman JD: The frequency of carcinoma and intraepithelial neoplasia of the prostate in young male patients. J Urol 150:379-385,1993.
3. Greenwald P and Lieberman R: Chemoprevention trials for prostate cancer. In: Chung L, Isaacs W and Simons J (eds): Prostate Cancer in the Twenty-First Century. Humana Press Inc, Totowa, NJ 2001, pp 499-518.
4. Kelloff GJ, Lieberman R, Brawer MK, Crawford ED and Miller G: Strategies for chemoprevention of prostate cancer. Prostate Cancer and Prostate Dis 2:27-33, 1999.
5. Tsai, H., Werber, J., Davia, M. O., Edelman, M., Tanaka, K. E., Melman, A., Christ, G.J., and Geliebter, J. Reduced connexin 43 expression in high grade, human prostatic adenocarcinoma cells. Biochem. Biophys. Res. Commun., *22:* 64-69,1996.
6. Mehta, P. P., Lokeshwar, B. L., Schiller, P. C., Bendix, M. V., Ostenson, R. C., Howard, G. A., and Roos, B. A. Gap-junctional communication in normal and neoplastic prostate epithelial cells and its regulation by cAMP. Mol. Carcinog., *15:* 18-32, 1996.
7. Mehta, P., Perez-Stable, C., Nadji, M., Mian, M., Asotra, K., and Roos, B. A. Suppression of human prostate cancer cell growth by forced expression of connexin genes. Develop. Gene., *24:* 91-110, 1999.
8. Mehta, P. P., Bertram, J. S., and Loewenstein, W. R. The actions of retinoids on cellular growth correlate with their actions on gap junctional communication. Cell Biol., *108:* 1053-1065, 1989.
9. Hossain MZ, Wilkens LR, Mehta PP, Loewenstein W, Bertram JS. Enhancement of gap junctional communication by retinoids correlates with their ability to inhibit neoplastic transformation. Carcinogenesis. 10:1743-1748, 1989.
10. Zhang, L. - X., Cooney, R. V., and Bertram, J. S. Carotenoids up-regulate connexin43 gene expression independent of their pro-vitamin A or antioxidant properties. Cancer Res., *52:* 5707-5712, 1992.
11. Rogers M, Berestecky JM, Hossain MZ, Guo HM, Kadle R, Nicholson BJ, Bertram JS. Retinoid-enhanced gap junctional communication is achieved by increased levels of connexin 43 mRNA and protein. Mol Carcinog. 3:335-343, 1990.
12. Goldberg GS, Bertram JS. Retinoids, gap junctional communication and suppression of epithelial tumors. In Vivo. 1994 8:745-754, 1994.
13. 13. Zhang, L. - X., Cooney, R. V., and Bertram, J. S. Carotenoids enhance gap junctional communication and inhibit lipid peroxidation in C3H/10T1/2 cells: Relationship to their cancer chemopreventive action. Carcinogenesis, *12:* 2109-2114, 1991.
14. Bertram, J. S., Pung, A., Churley, M., Kappock, T. J. 4th, Wilkins, L. R, and Cooney, R. V. Diverse carotenoids protect against chemically induced neoplastic transformation. Carcinogenesis, *12:* 671-678, 1991.
15. Rajah, R., Valentinis, B., and Cohen, P. Insulin-like growth factor (IGF)-binding protein-3 induces apoptosis and mediates the effects of transforming growth factor-beta-1 on programmed cell death through a p53- and IGF-independent mechanism. J. Biol. Chem., *272:* 12181-12188, 1997.
16. Cohen, P., Peehl, D.M., and Rosenfeld, R.G. The IGF axis in the prostate. Hormone Metab. Res., *26:* 81-84, 1994.
17. Cohen, P., Peehl, D.M., Lamson, G., and Rosenfeld, R.G. Insulin-like growth factors (IGFs), IGF receptors, and IGF-binding proteins in primary cultures of prostate epithelial cells. J. Clin. Endocrinol. Metab., *73:* 401-407, 1991.
18. Chan, J. M., Stampfer, M. J., Giovanucci, E., Gann, P. H., Ma, J., Wilkinson, P.,

Hennekens, C. H., and Pollak, M. Plasma insulin-like growth factor-1 and prostate cancer risk: a prospective study. Science, *279:* 563-566, 1998.

19. Giovannucci, E. Insulin-like growth factor-I and binding protein-3 and risk of cancer. Horm. Res., *51 (Suppl 3):* 34-41, 1999.
20. Mantzoros, C. S., Tzonou, A., Signorello, L. B., Stampfer, M., Trichopoulos, D., and Adami, H. O. Insulin-like growth factor-1 in relation to prostate cancer and benign prostatic hyperplasia. Br. J. Cancer, *76:* 1115-1118, 1997.
21. Wolk, A., Mantzoros, C. S., Andersson, S. O., Bergstrom, R., Signorello, L. B., Lagiou, P., Adami, H. O., and Trichopoulos, D. Insulin-like growth factor-1 and prostate cancer risk: a population-based, case-control study. J. Natl. Cancer Inst., *90:* 911-915, 1998.
22. Pollak, M., Beamer, W., and Zhang, J. C. Insulin-like growth factors and prostate cancer. Cancer Met. Rev., *17:* 383-390, 1998-99.
23. Sharoni Y, Levy Y, et al. Personal communication and unpublished observations.
24. Giovannucci, E., and Clinton, S. K. Tomatoes, lycopene, and prostate cancer. Proc. Soc. Exp.Biol. Med., *218:* 129-139, 1998.
25. Gann P. H., Ma, J., Giovannucci, E., Willett, W., Sacks, F. M., Hennekens, C. H., and Stampfer,M. J. Lower prostate cancer risk in men with elevated plasma lycopene levels: results of a prospective analysis. Cancer Res., *59:* 1225-1230, 1999.
26. Giovannucci, E. Tomatoes, tomato-based products, lycopene, and cancer: review of the epidemiologic literature. J. Natl. Cancer Inst., *91:* 317-331, 1999.
27. Giovannucci, E., Aschorio, A., Rimm, E. B., Stampfer, M. J., Colditz, G. A., and Willett, W. C. Intake of carotenoids and retinol in relation to risk of prostate cancer. J. Natl. Cancer Inst., *87:* 1767-1776, 1995.
28. Kelloff, G. J., Lieberman, R., Steele, V. E., Boone, C. W., Lubet, R. A., Kopelovitch, L., Malone, W. A., Crowell, J. A., and Sigman, C. C. Chemoprevention of prostate cancer: concepts and strategies. Euro. Urol., *35:* 342-350, 1999.
29. Bertram, J.S. Carotenoids and gene regulation. Nutrition Rev. *57*:182-191, 1999.
30. Amir, H., Karas, M., Giat, J., Danilenko, M., Levy, R., Yermiahu, T., Levy, J., and Sharoni, Y. Lycopene and 1,25-dihydroxyvitamin D3 cooperate in the inhibition of cell cycle progression and induction of differentiation in HL-60 leukemic cells. Nutr. Cancer, *33:* 105-112,1999.
31. Levy, J., Bosin, E., Feldman, B., Giat, Y., Miinster, A., Danilenko, M., and Sharoni, Y. Lycopene is a more potent inhibitor of human cancer cell proliferation than either alpha-carotene or beta-carotene. Nutr. Cancer, *24:* 257-266, 1995.
32. Park, C. K., Ishimi, Y., Ohmura, M., Yamaguchi, M., and Ikegami, S. Vitamin A and carotenoids stimulate differentiation of mouse osteoblastic cells. J. Nutr. Sci. Vitaminol., *43:* 281-296, 1997.
33. Karas, M., Amir, H., Fishman, D., Danilenko, M., Segal, S., Nahum, A., Koifmann, A., Giat, Y., Levy, J., and Sharoni, Y. Lycopene interferes with cell cycle progression and insulin-like growth factor I signaling in mammary cancer cells. Nutr. Cancer, *36:* 101-111, 2000.
34. Nickerson, T., Pollak, M., and Huynh, H. Castration-induced apoptosis in the rat ventral prostate is associated with increased expression of genes encoding insulin-like growth factor binding proteins 2,3,4 and 5. Endocrinology, *139:* 807-810,1998.
35. Miyake, H., Pollak, M., and Gleave, M. E. Castration-induced up-regulation of insulin-like growth factor binding protein-5 potentiates insulin-like growth factor-I activity and accelerates progression to androgen independence in prostate cancer models. Cancer Res., *60:* 3058-3064, 2000.

36. Rajah, R., Khare, A., Lee, P. D., and Cohen, P. Insulin-like growth factor-binding protein-3 is partially responsible for high-serum-induced apoptosis in PC-3 prostate cancer cells. J. Endocrinol., *163:* 487-494, 1999.
37. Matsushima-Nishiwaki, R., Shidoji, Y., Nishiwaki, S., Yamada, T., Moriwaki, H., and Muto, Y. Suppression by carotenoids of microcystin-induced morphological changes in mouse hepatocytes. Lipids, *30:* 1029-1034, 1995.
38. Hotz-Wagenblatt, A., and Shalloway, D. Gap junctional communication and neoplastic transformation. Crit. Rev. Oncogenesis, *4:* 541-558, 1993.
39. Bertram, J. S., and Bortkiewicz, H. Dietary carotenoids inhibit neoplastic transformation and modulate gene expression in mouse and human cells. Am. J. Clin. Nutr., *62 (6 suppl):* 1327s-1336s, 1995.
40. Beyer, E. C., Paul, D. L., and Goodenough, D. A. Connexin43: a protein from rat heart homologous to a gap junction protein from liver. J. Cell Biol., *105:* 2621-2629, 1987.
41. Mehta, P. P., Bertram, J. S., and Loewenstein, W. R. Growth inhibition of transformed cells correlates with their junctional communication with normal cells. Cell, *44:* 187-196, 1986.
42. Loewenstein, W. R. Junctional intercellular communication and the control of growth. Biochem. Biophys. Acta, *560:* 1-65, 1979.
43. Yamasaki, H. Gap junctional intercellular communication and carcinogenesis. Carcinogenesis, *11:* 1051-1058, 1990.
44. Chen, S. - C., Pelletier, D. B., Peng, A., and Boynton, A. L. Connexin43 reverses the phenotype of transformed cells and alters their expression of cyclin/cyclin-dependent kinases. Cell Growth Diff., *6:* 681-690, 1995.
45. Gius, D., Botero, A., Shah, S., and Curry, H. A. Intracellular oxidation/reduction status in the regulation of transcription factors NF-kappaB and AP-1. Toxicol. Lett., *106:* 93-106, 1999.
46. Riso, P., Pinder, A., Santangelo, A., and Porrini, M. Does tomato consumption effectively increase the resistance of lymphocyte DNA to oxidative damage? Am. J. Clin. Nutr., *69:* 712-718, 1999.
47. Rao, A.V., Fleshner, N., and Agarwal, S. Serum and tissue lycopene and biomarkers of oxidation in prostate cancer patients: a case-control study. Nutr. Cancer, *33:* 159-64, 1999.
48. Jewell, C., and O'Brien, N. M. Effect of dietary supplementation with carotenoids on xenobiotic metabolizing enzymes in the liver, lung, kidney and small intestine of the rat. Br. J. Nutr., *81:* 235-242, 1999.
49. Conn, P. F., Schlach, W., and Truscott, T. G. The singlet oxygen and carotenoid interaction [published erratum appears in J. Photochem. Photobiol. B, *17:* 89, 1993]. J. Photochem. Photobiol. *11:* 41-47, 1991.
50. DiMascio, P., Kaiser, S., and Sies, H. Lycopene as the most efficient biological carotenoid singlet oxygen quencher. Arch. Biochem. Biophys., *274:* 1-7, 1989.
51. Clinton, S. K., Emenhiser, C., Schwartz, S. J., Bostwick, D. G., Williams, A. W., Moore, B. J., and Erdman, J. W. Jr. Cis-trans lycopene isomers, carotenoids and retinol in human prostate. Cancer Epidemiol. Biomarkers Prev., *5:* 823-833, 1996.
52. Rao, A. V., and Agarwal, S. Bioavailability and in vivo antioxidant properties of lycopene from tomato products and their possible role in the prevention of cancer. Nutr. Cancer, *31:* 199-203, 1998.
53. Rao, A. V., Fleshner, N., and Agarwal, S. Serum and tissue lycopene and biomarkers of oxidation in prostate cancer patients: A case-control study. Nutr. Cancer, *33:* 159-164, 1999.

54. Kucuk O, Sarkar F, Sakr W, Djuric Z, Khachik F, Pollak M, Bertram J, Grignon D, Banerjee M, Crissman J, Pontes E, Wood DP Jr. Phase II randomized clinical trial of lycopene supplementation before radical prostatectomy. Cancer Epidemiol Biomarkers Prev 10:861-868, 2001.
55. Sakr, W. A. Prostatic intraepithelial neoplasia: A marker for high-risk groups and a potential target for chemoprevention. Eur. Urol., *35:* 474-478, 1999.
56. Chen L, Stazewicz-Sapuntzakis M, Duncan C, Sharifi R, Ghosh L, vanBreemen R, Ashton D, Bowen PE. Oxidative DNA damage in prostate cancer patients consuming tomato sauce-based entrees as a whole-food intervention. J Natl Can Inst 93(24):1872-9, 2001.
57. Ansari MS, Gupta NP. A comparison of lycopene and orchidectomy vs orchidectomy alone in the management of advanced prostate cancer. BJU International 92(4):375-8, 2003.
58. He, Y., and Campbell, T. C. Effects of carotenoids on aflatoxin B1-induced mutagenesis in S. typhimurium TA 100 and TA 98. Nutr. Cancer, *13:* 243-253, 1990.
59. Bertram, J. S. Cancer prevention by carotenoids. In: L. M. Canfield, N. I. Krinsky, and J. A. Olson (eds). Carotenoids in Health, V.691, pp177-191. Ann. N. Y. Acad. Sci., NY, 1993.
60. Nishino H. Cancer prevention by natural carotenoids. J. Cell. Biochem., *27(Suppl):* 86-91,1997.
61. Neveu, M., and Bertram, J. S. Gap junctions and neoplasia. In Gap Junctions, Hetzberg, E. L. and Bittar, E. E. (eds). JAI Press, Greenwich, CT, pp 221-262, 2000.
62. Jones, J. I., and Clemmons D. R. Insulin-like growth factors and their binding proteins: biological actions. Endocr. Rev., *16:* 3-34, 1995.
63. Lee, S. W., Tomasetto, C., and Sager, R. Positive selection of candidate tumor suppressor genes by subtractive hybridization. Proc. Natl. Acad. Sci. USA, *88:* 2825-2829, 1991.
64. Omori,Y. and H.Yamasaki: Mutated connexin43 proteins inhibit rat glioma cell growth suppression mediated by wild-type connexin43 in a dominant- negative manner. Int. J. Cancer, *78:* 446-453, 1998.
65. Hossain, M.Z., and Bertram, J. S. Retinoids suppress proliferation, induce cell spreading, and up-regulate connexin43 expression only in postconfluent 10T1/2 cells: Implications for the role of gap junctional communication. Cell Growth Diff., *5:* 1253-1261, 1994.
66. King, T. J., Fukushima, L. H., Hieber, A. D., Shimabukuro, K. A., Sakr, W. A., and Bertram, J. S. Reduced levels of connexin 43 in cervical dysplasia: inducible expression in a cervical carcinoma cell line decreases neoplastic potential with implications for tumor progression. Carcinogenesis, *21:* 1097-1109, 2000.
67. Hossain, M. Z., Jagdale, A. B., Ao, P., LeCiel, C., Huang, R. P., and Boynton, A. L. Impaired expression and posttranslational processing of connexin 43 and downregulation of gap junctional communication in neoplastic human prostate cells. Prostate, 38:55-59,1999.

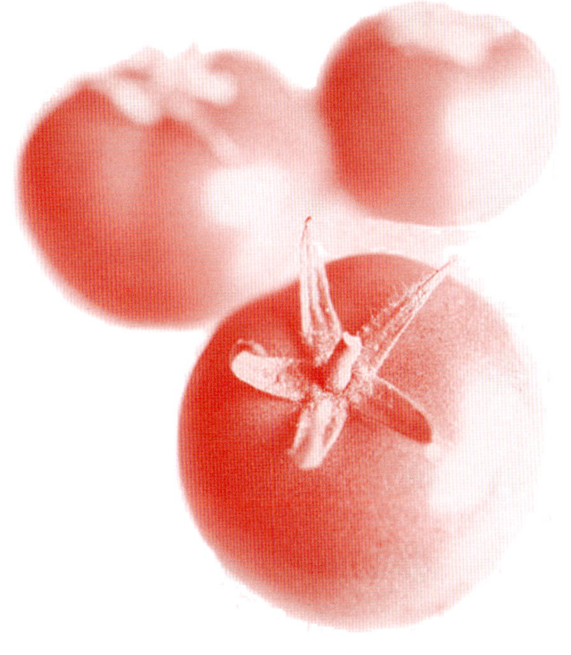

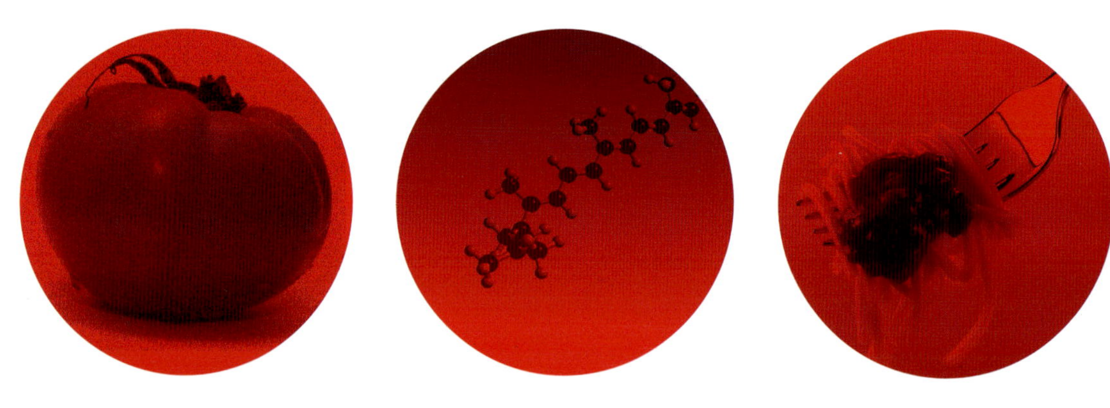

Lycopene and Cardiovascular Disease

Dr.Tiina Rissanen
Research Institute of Public Health,
School of Public Health and Clinical Nutrition
University of Kuopio, Finland

Abstract

Diets rich in fruits and vegetables have aroused interest because of their potential health benefits against chronic diseases, such as cardiovascular diseases (CVD) and cancer.

CVD are a major global public health problem, representing the most common cause of death in Europe and in many industrialized countries. There are likely to be multiple mechanisms through which a plant-dominated diet can protect against CVD. The proposed beneficial substances include many components including carotenoids. Although carotenoids are not essential for human health, they have biological actions that may be important in maintaining health and preventing chronic diseases such as CVD. This review summarizes the major findings of CVD-related epidemiologic research on lycopene.

INTRODUCTION

Cardiovascular diseases (CVD) are a major global public health problem, representing the most common cause of death in Europe and in many industrialized countries (1). For example, in the USA, coronary heart disease (CHD) was responsible for nearly 500,000 deaths in 2002 (2). However the CVD prevalence rate varies greatly between national populations. In the Seven Countries Study (3), low coronary heart disease (CHD) -related mortality rates have been found in southern European countries and Japan in contrast to the high mortality rates that have been found in the USA, the Netherlands and Finland. Nutrition plays an important role in the development of CVD and diets also vary extensively between different populations. In the eastern part of Finland, the mortality rate was 10-times higher than in Crete where the population consumes a Mediterranean diet rich in plant foods year-round and relatively poor in animal foods (3). There are likely to be multiple mechanisms through which a plant-dominated diet can promote health. Carotenoids, especially lycopene, are one of many proposed beneficial substances. Although carotenoids are not essential for human health, they have biological actions that may be important in maintaining health and preventing chronic diseases such as CVD.

Very little is known about the specific biological mechanisms through which lycopene and other carotenoids can protect against atherosclerosis and CVD. However, many of the biological effects and health benefits of carotenoids are hypothesized to occur via protection against oxidative damage (4). Alterations in acute phase response in atherosclerosis might be one mechanism through which lycopene exerts its protective effect. Lycopene is the only carotenoid which can reduce both the monocyte adhesion of the human aortic endothelial cell and the expression of adhesion molecules on the cell surface (5). Intracellular gap junction communication, hormonal and immune system modulation are pathways through which lycopene could also inhibit atherosclerosis (4,6).

EPIDEMIOLOGICAL EVIDENCE ABOUT LYCOPENE, ATHEROSCLEROSIS, AND CARDIOVASCULAR DISEASES

The association between dietary intake or blood or tissue concentration of lycopene and CVD and atherosclerosis has been studied over the last ten years (Table1 p.146). One of the first reports to suggest a possible relationship between lycopene and CVD risk was the nested case-control study published in 1994 by Street and co-workers (7). This American nested case-control study examined the association between serum levels of carotenoids and subsequent myocardial infarction in 123 cases and 246 controls. During a 14 year follow up, they found an increased risk of events in smokers with lower serum levels of ß-carotene, lycopene, lutein and zeaxanthin, but not in nonsmokers. In 1997, Kristenson and co-workers published results from the cross-sectional Linköping-Vilnus Coronary Risk Assessment Study (8). There were lower plasma levels of lycopene, ß-carotene and α-tocopherol and a higher CHD mortality in Lithuania as compared to Sweden. In addition, the authors found a difference in oxidation of LDL between these two populations and suggested that the increase in CHD in Lithuania may be related to the lower antioxidant status of that population.

The multicenter case-control European Study of Antioxidants, Myocardial Infarction and Cancer of the Breast (EURAMIC) examined the association between the antioxidant concentration in fat tissue and the incidence of myocardial infarction in ten countries (9). The study found that men with the highest concentrations of lycopene in their adipose tissue had a 48% reduction in the risk of developing CVD when compared with those men with the lowest lycopene levels. In a part of the same EURAMIC study from the Malaga center (10), there was a 60% lower risk of myocardial infarction among those participants in the highest fifth of adipose tissue lycopene concentration as compared with the participants in the lowest fifth.

In the Finnish prospective Kuopio Ischaemic Heart Disease Risk Factor (KIHD) study involving 1038 middle-aged men, serum levels of lycopene were inversely and independently associated with the risk-acute coronary event or stroke [RR 3.3 (95% Confidence Interval (CI) 1.7 to 6.4) for the lowest quarter compared with the three other quarters] (11). In this study, 12.6% of men in the lowest quarter and 3.3 % in other quarters suffered an acute coronary event or stroke during the follow-up time of 5.3 years. The protective effect remained during a longer follow-up of 7.6 years (12).

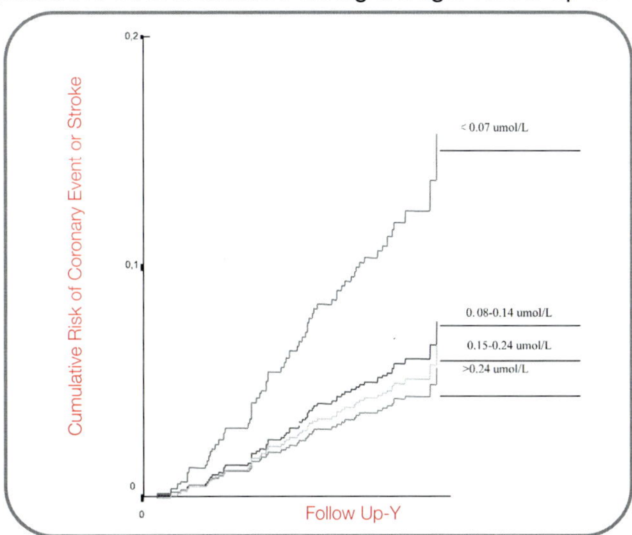

Fig 1: Cumulative morbidity of an acute coronary event or a stroke occurring during follow-up 9 years and 10 months according to the quarters of the serum concentration of lycopene in middle aged Finnish men in the KIHD study (Rissanen 2003).

In the Physicians' Health Study, Hak and co-workers prospectively examined the association between plasma levels of five major carotenoids, including lycopene, and stroke and myocardial infarction (13,14). Men with high plasma levels of lycopene (2-5 fifth), had a 39% (CI 0 to 63%) decreased risk of stroke as compared with men whose plasma lycopene levels were in the lowest fifth. However they did not find any protective association between the plasma carotenoids and the myocardial infarction risk. Recently the same Physicians' Health Study reported no association between plasma lycopene levels or other carotenoids and CVD among older and middle-aged men (15). In the prospective Women's Health Study, Sesso and colleagues studied prospectively the association between plasma levels of lycopene and other carotenoids and the risk of CVD (16). The women with plasma levels of lycopene greater than the median had a 34% (95% CI 5 to 53%) decreased risk of CVD compared with the others. They also noted an L-shaped association between increasing quartiles of plasma levels of lycopene and the lower risk of CVD in middle-aged and older women. In a Costa Rican case-control study, there were inverse associations between lycopene levels of adipose tissue and acute myocardial infarction, however the associations did not remain significant after adjustments for other confounding factors(17).

The prevalence of carotid plaques and increased thickness of the intima media have been shown to predict coronary events and therefore have been claimed to represent an early stage of atherogenesis (18). In an American case-control study performed by the participants in the Atherosclerosis Risk in Communities (ARIC) study (19), an increase in the serum concentration of lycopene was associated with nonsignificantly lower odds of being a case (the 90th percentile of IMT) after adjusting for other CVD risk factors. In 2000, D'Odorico and colleague published cross-sectional and prospective data from the Bruneck study; high plasma levels of α- and ß-carotene but not lycopene were associated with a decreased 5-year incidence of atherosclerotic lesions in the carotid arteries (20). In contrast, in the Dutch Rotterdam Study, Klipstein-Grobusch and co-workers observed that serum lycopene was the only carotenoid which was associated with decreased risk of aortic atherosclerosis in current and former smokers after adjusting for age and sex (21). A similar but nonsignificant association was seen among the whole study population. The inverse association between lycopene levels and carotid intima media thickness (IMT) among smokers was also seen in the Los Angeles Atherosclerosis Study (22). However the relationship was not significant among the whole study population.

The Antioxidant Supplementation in Atherosclerosis Prevention (ASAP) study examined cardiovascular risk factors and intake of nutrients in Finnish men and women. After adjustment for other risk factors a low level of plasma lycopene was associated with a 17.8% increment in intima media thickness of common carotid artery (CCA-IMT) in men (23). An inverse association was also seen among women but the difference did not remain statistically significant after the adjustments. Similarly lower blood levels of lycopene were also found to be associated with increased IMT in another Finnish study. In the KIHD study the association between serum levels of lycopene and carotid atherosclerosis was studied in 1028 eastern Finnish men (24). Low serum levels of lycopene were associated with a significant increment in CCA-IMT. Both the mean and maximal CCA-IMT increased linearly across the quarters of serum levels of lycopene. McQuillan and co-workers examined the relationship between antioxidants including lycopene and carotid atherosclerosis in the Australian Carotid Ultrasound Disease Assessment Study (CUDAS) (25). They found an inverse association between CCA-IMT and plasma lycopene in women but not in men. A small Italian study pointed to a trend that those participants with essential hypertension and peripheral vascular disease had a lower plasma lycopene level than healthy subjects or participants with uncomplicated hypertension (26). Serum lycopene also showed a statistical significantly negative correlation with maximal IMT.

The association between dietary intake of lycopene and CVD has been studied only in a few studies. In the prospective Health Professionals' Study (27), a high dietary intake of lutein was associated with a reduced risk for ischemic stroke, whereas the dietary intake of lycopene or α- or ß-carotene measured by a food-frequency questionnaire showed no association with the stroke risk. In the ATBC study which examined a total of 26,593 smokers, dietary lycopene was inversely associated with the risk of cerebral infarction and subarachnoid hemorrhage [RRs 0.74 (95% CI 0.59 to 0.92) and 0.39 (95% CI 0.21 to 0.74), respectively]. Negative relationships were also noted between beta-carotene and cerebral infarction and lutein plus zeaxanthin and subarachnoid hemorrhage (28). The association between dietary carotenoids and coronary artery diseases was studied in the Nurses' Health Study (29) where there was a modest inverse association between coronary artery diseases and alpha- and beta-carotene levels, but not for lycopene, lutein plus zeaxantin or beta-cryptoxanthin concentrations in women. In the Women's Health Study, there were weak and nonsignificant inverse associations between dietary intake of lycopene and cardiovascular diseases (30). However, in that study, high intake of tomato-based foodstuffs seemed to be associated with a reduced risk of CVD. The recent pooled analysis from the Pooling Project of Cohort Studies on Diet and Coronary Disease did not find any association between energy-adjusted dietary intake of lycopene and CHD (31).

Study, nationality of subjects	Type of study Follow-up (years)	Sex	n	Outcome
American (Street et al. 1994)	Nested case-control 14 years	F, M	123 + 246	MI
ARIC study American (Iribarren et al. 1997)	Case-control	F, M	462	IMT
The Linköping-Vilnus Coronary Disease Risk Assessment study, Swedish, Lithuanian(Kristenson et al. 1997)	Cross sectional		210	CHD mortality
EURAMIC study, Multicenter (Kohlmeier et al. 1997)	Case-control	M	1,379	MI
The Health Professionals Follow-up Study American (Ascherio et al. 1999)	Prospective 8 years	M	43,738	Stroke
ATBC Study Finnish, (Hirvonen et al. 2000)	Prospective 6.1 years	M	26,953	Stroke
The Rotterdan study Dutch , (Klipstein-Grobusch et al. 2000)	Case-control	F, M	108 + 108	Plaques of the abdominal aorta
Bruneck study Italian, (D'Odorico et al. 2000)	Cross sectional and prospective 5 years	F, M	392	Prevalence and incidence of carotid plaques
ASAP Study Finnish, (Rissanen et al. 2000)	Cross sectional	F, M	520	IMT
The CUDAS study Australian, (McQuillan et al. 2001)	Cross sectional	F, M	1,111	IMT
KIHD study Finnish, (Rissanen et al. 2001)	Cross sectional	M	1,028	IMT
KIHD study Finnish, (Rissanen et al. 2001), (Rissanen 2003)	Prospective 5.3 years, 7.6 years	M	725	MI, stroke
Italian (Gianetti et al. 2002)	Case-control	F,M	33	IMT
Physicians' Health Study American, (Hak et al. 2003)	Nested case-control 13 years	M	531+531	MI
Nurses Health Study American. (Osganian et al. 2003)	Prospective 12 years	F	73,286	CAD
Womens' Health Study American, Sesso et al. 2003)	Prospective 7.2 years	F	39,876	CVD
The Los Angeles Atherosclerosis study American, (Dwyer et al. 2004)	Cohort 1.5 years	F, M	573	IMT
Physicians' Health Study American, (Hak et al. 2004),	Nested case-control 13 years	M	297+297	Stroke
Womens' Health Study American, (Sesso et al. 2004),	Nested case-control 4.8 years	F	483 + 483	CVD
Physicians' Health Study American, (Sesso et al. 2005)	Nested case-control 2.1 years	M	499 + 499	CVD
Costa Rican (Kabagambe et al. 2005)	Case-control	F, M	1,456 + 1,456	MI

Table 1: Studies on the association of lycopene with the risk of CVD and atherosclerosis.

Source of lycopene	Main Results
Serum	63% lower risk of MI among smokers with low level s of lycopene.
Serum	Nonsignificantly lower odds of being a case with increases in lycopene.
Plasma	Lower levels of lycopene and higher risk of CHD mortality in Vilnus than in Link ping
Adipose tissue	48% lower risk of MI in the highest 10th percentile lycopene as the others.
Dietary intake	No association between the risk of stroke and dietary intake of lycopene.
Dietary intake	Dietary lycopene was inversely associated with the risk for cerebral infarction and subarachnoid hemorrhage.
Serum	An inverse association between high lycopene levels and the risk of atherosclerosis among current and former smokers.
Serum	Lycopene did not significantly predict against the risk of atherosclerosis.
Plasma	Low plasma lycopene levels were associated with early atherosclerosis in men.
Plasma	An inverse association between plasma lycopene and CC-IMT in women.
Serum	Low levels of lycopene are associated with higher mean and maximal CCA-IMT
Serum	3.3 times higher risk of acute coronary event or stroke among participants with low levels of lycopene. Protective effect remains during longer follow-up.
Plasma	An inverse association between lycopene and IMT in patients with essential hypertension and peripheral vascular diseases compared with healthy controls and patients with uncomplicated hypertension.
Plasma	Lycopene did not predict against the risk of MI.
Dietary intake	No association between dietary lycopene and CAD.
Dietary intake	Lycopene did not significantly predict against the risk of CVD.
Plasma	Lycopene was protective against progression of IMT among smokers.
Plasma	Nonsignificantly lower risk of ischemic stroke among men with high levels of lycopene.
Plasma	34% decreased risk of CVD among participants in upper compared the lower half of plasma lycopene. 50% decreased risk of CVD (exlusive of angina) among women in the upper 3 quartiles compared with the lowest quartile.
Plasma	No association between lycopene and CVD in older men.
Adipose tissue	Lycopene did not predict against the risk of MI.

CHD= coronary heart disease, CVD= cardiovascular diseases, CAD= coronary artery disease, MI= myocardial infarction, CCA-IMT= intima media thickness of carotid artery wall, IMT= intima media thickness F=female, M= male.

Table 1: Studies on the association of lycopene with the risk of CVD and atherosclerosis.

SUMMARY

The evidence emerging from the epidemiological studies is compatible with a protective action of lycopene on CVD, but it is still open to discussion overall. Sixteen studies have reported an inverse association between circulating or tissue levels or dietary intake of lycopene and atherosclerosis or CVD, but six studies and in addition one meta-analysis reported no such association. However, in some of the studies, an inverse association between lycopene and CVD was seen in certain subgroups of the study population. The mean blood concentration of lycopene has varied extensively in population-based studies from European countries and the USA (8, 15, 20, 21, 23-25). The most likely explanation for this variation is the difference in the dietary intake of tomatoes or tomato products between populations. In the United Kingdom and Finland, the daily intake of lycopene has been 1 mg/day or lower, whereas in the USA and Ireland eight to ten times higher intakes have been described (28, 32-34). In 1984-89, in the baseline part of the Finnish KIHD study, over 40% of the population did not consume any lycopene during the four-day food recording (12). In many countries it may be difficult to find subjects with very low circulating levels of lycopene, and low range in values could be one explanation for the weak association described in some studies.

Another explanation could be that there is a threshold effect for lycopene levels. In the Women's Health Study the association between the plasma level of lycopene and the risk of CVD appeared to be L-shaped (16). A similar but weaker L-shaped association between plasma lycopene and ischemic stroke was seen in the Physicians' Health Study (14). Similarly, in the KIHD study, men in the lowest quarter of serum levels of lycopene had an over three times higher risk of an acute coronary event or stroke as compared with the others (Figure 1).

Thirdly, it is possible that the serum levels of lycopene could simply represent an indicator or surrogate for some other beneficial dietary or lifestyle factors. However, the correlation between blood lycopene concentrations and total intake of vegetables and fruits has been previously shown to be very low (35). Thus blood lycopene may not simply be a reflection of a healthy diet. Lycopene is found mainly in tomatoes and tomato products. Other sources of lycopene are watermelon, rosehips, pink grapefruit and guava (36, 37). The total intake of vegetables and fruits is known to be the most significant determinant for plasma carotenoids except for lycopene and thus blood carotenoid levels are useful biomarkers of vegetables and fruits intake (35). In the NHANES III (38), there was a significant positive association between the intake of fruits and vegetables and the concentrations of carotenoids, but not for lycopene. Tomatoes account for over 80% of the lycopene in the American diet (38). In northern European countries, consumption of tomatoes may account for even greater proportions.

CONCLUSION

The findings from epidemiological studies support the claim that higher blood or tissue levels of lycopene or higher intake of lycopene from dietary sources are beneficial in the prevention of atherosclerosis and CVD. However, there are still many questions concerning the role of lycopene and tomato products in cardiovascular health and more studies will be needed to clarify this association. In addition, a large intervention study would help to evaluate the relation between the intake of lycopene (or tomatoes and tomato products) and the risk of CVD.

REFERENCES:

1. Fact sheet EURO 2004. Internet: http://www.euro.who.int/. (accessed 4. September 2005).
2. Cardiovascular Disease Statistics 2005. American Heart Association. Internet: http://www.americanheart.org. (accessed 2. September 2005).
3. Menotti A, Kromhout D, Blackburn H, Fidanza F, Buzina R and Nissinen A. Food intake patterns and 25-year mortality from coronary heart disease: cross-cultural correlations in the Seven Countries Study. The Seven Countries Study Research Group. Eur J Epidemiol 1999;15:507-515.
4. Tapiero H, Townsend DM, Tew KD. The role of carotenoids in the prevention of human pathologies. Biomed Pharmacother. 2004;58:100-110.
5. Martin KR, Wu D and Meydani M. The effect of carotenoids on the expression of cell surface adhesion molecules and binding of monocytes to human aortic endothelial cells. Atherosclerosis 2000;150:265-274.
6. Rao AV, Agarwal S. Am Coll Nutr. Role of antioxidant lycopene in cancer and heart disease. 2000;19:563-569.
7. Street DA, Comstock GW, Salkeld RM, Schuep W and Klag MJ. Serum antioxidants and myocardial infarction. Are low levels of carotenoids and alpha-tocopherol risk factors for myocardial infarction? Circulation 1994;90:1154-1161.
8. Kristenson M, Zieden B, Kucinskiene Z, Elinder LS, Bergdahl B, Elwing B, Abaravicius A, Razinkoviene L, Calkauskas H and Olsson AG. Antioxidant state and mortality from coronary heart disease in Lithuanian and Swedish men: concomitant cross sectional study of men aged 50. BMJ 1997;314:629-633.
9. Kohlmeier L, Kark JD, Gomez-Gracia E, Martin BC, Steck SE, Kardinaal AF, Ringstad J, Thamm M, Masaev V, Riemersma R, Martin-Moreno JM, Huttunen JK and Kok FJ. Lycopene and myocardial infarction risk in the EURAMIC Study. Am J Epidemiol 1997;146:618-626.

10. Gomez-Aracena J, Sloots J and Garcia-Rodriguez A. Antioxidants in adipose tissue and myocardial infarction in a Mediterranean area. The EURAMIC study in Malaga. Nutr Metab Cardiovasc Dis 1997;:376-377-382.
11. Rissanen T, Voutilainen S, Nyyssönen K, Lakka TA, Salonen R, Kaplan GA, Salonen JT. Low serum lycopene is associated with excess risk of acute coronary events and stroke: The Kuopio Ischaemic Risk Factor Study. Brit J Nutr 2001;85:749-754.
12. Rissanen T. Association of lycopene and dietary intake of fruits, berries and vegetables with atherosclerosis and cardiovascular diseases. Epidemiologic evidence. Kuopio University Publications D. Medical Sciences 304. Kuopio University Printing Office. Kuopio 2003. Finland.
13. Hak AE, Stampfer MJ, Campos H, Sesso HD, Gaziano JM, Willett W, Ma J. Plasma carotenoids and tocopherols and risk of myocardial infarction in a low-risk population of US male physicians. Circulation. 2003;108:802-807.
14. Hak AE, Ma J, Powell CB, Campos H, Gaziano JM, Willett WC, Stampfer MJ. Prospective study of plasma carotenoids and tocopherols in relation to risk of ischemic stroke. Stroke. 2004;35:1584-1588.
15. Sesso HD, Buring JE, Norkus EP, Gaziano JM. Plasma lycopene, other carotenoids, and retinol and the risk of cardiovascular disease in men. Am J Clin Nutr. 2005;81:990-997.
16. Sesso HD, Buring JE, Norkus EP, Gaziano JM. Plasma lycopene, other carotenoids, and retinol and the risk of cardiovascular disease in women. Am J Clin Nutr. 2004; 79:47-53.
17. Kabagambe EK, Furtado J, Baylin A, Campos H. Some dietary and adipose tissue carotenoids are associated with the risk of nonfatal acute myocardial infarction in Costa Rica. J Nutr. 2005;135:1763-1769.
18. Salonen JT, Salonen R. Ultrasonographically assessed carotid morphology and the risk of coronary heart disease. Arterioscler Thromb. 1991;11:1245–1249.
19. Iribarren C, Folsom AR, Jacobs DR, Gross MD, Belcher JD and Eckfeldt JH. Association of serum vitamin levels, LDL susceptibility to oxidation, and autoantibodies against MDA-LDL with carotid atherosclerosis. A case- control study. Arterioscler Thromb Vasc Biol 1997;17:1171-1177.
20. D'Odorico A, Martines D, Kiechl S, Egger G, Oberhollenzer F, Bonvicini P, Sturniolo GC, Naccarato R and Willeit J. High plasma levels of alpha- and beta-carotene are associated with a lower risk of atherosclerosis: results from the Bruneck study. Atherosclerosis 2000;153:231-239.
21. Klipstein-Grobusch K, Launer LJ, Geleijnse JM, Boeing H, Hofman A and Witteman JC. Serum carotenoids and atherosclerosis. The Rotterdam Study. Atherosclerosis 2000;148:49-56.
22. Dwyer JH, Paul-Labrador MJ, Fan J, Shircore AM, Merz CN, Dwyer KM. Progression of carotid intima-media thickness and plasma antioxidants: the Los Angeles Atherosclerosis Study. Arterioscler Thromb Vasc Biol. 2004;24:313-319.
23. Rissanen T, Voutilainen S, Nyyssönen K, Salonen R, Salonen JT. Low plasma lycopene concentration is associated with increased intima-media thickness of the carotid artery wall. Arterioscler Thromb Vasc Biol 2000;20:2677-2681.
24. Rissanen T, Voutilainen S, Nyyssönen K, Salonen R, Kaplan GA, Salonen JT. Serum lycopene level and carotid atherosclerosis: the Kuopio Ischaemic Heart Disease Risk Factor (KIHD) Study. Am J Clin Nutr 2003;77:133-138.

25. McQuillan BM, Hung J, Beilby JP, Nidorf M and Thomson PL. Antioxidant Vitamins and the Risk of Carotid Atherosclerosis. Journal of American College of Cardiology 2001;38:1788-1794.
26. Gianetti J, Pedrinelli R, Petrucci R, Lazzerini G, De Caterina M, Bellomo G and De Caterina R. Inverse association between carotid intima-media thickness and the antioxidant lycopene in atherosclerosis. Am Heart J 2002;143:467-474.
27. Ascherio A, Rimm EB, Hernan MA, Giovannucci E, Kawachi I, Stampfer MJ and Willett WC. Relation of consumption of vitamin E, vitamin C, and carotenoids to risk for stroke among men in the United States. Ann Intern Med 1999;130:963-970.
28. Hirvonen T, Virtamo J, Korhonen P, Albanes D and Pietinen P. Intake of flavonoids, carotenoids, vitamins C and E, and risk of stroke in male smokers. Stroke 2000;31:2301-2306.
29. Osganian SK, Stampfer MJ, Rimm E, Spiegelman D, Manson JAE, Willett WC. Dietary carotenoids and risk of coronary artery disease in women. Am J Clin Nutr 2003;77:1390-1399.
30. Sesso HD, Liu S, Gaziano JM, Buring JE. Dietary lycopene, tomato-based food products and cardiovascular disease in women. J Nutr. 2003;133:2336-2341.
31. Knekt P, Ritz J, Pereira MA, O'Reilly EJ, Augustsson K, Fraser GE, Goldbourt U, Heitmann BL, Hallmans G, Liu S, Pietinen P, Spiegelman D, Stevens J, Virtamo J, Willett WC, Rimm EB, Ascherio A. Antioxidant vitamins and coronary heart disease risk: a pooled analysis of 9 cohorts. Am J Clin Nutr. 2004;80:1508-1520.
32. Järvinen R. Carotenoids, retinoids, tocopherols and tocotrienols in the diet; the Finnish Mobile Clinic Health Examination Survey. Int J Vitam Nutr Res 1995;65:24-30.
33. Slattery ML, Benson J, Curtin K, Ma KN, Schaeffer D and Potter JD. Carotenoids and colon cancer. Am J Clin Nutr 2000;71:575-582.
34. Porrini M, Riso P. What are typical lycopene intakes? J Nutr. 2005;135:2042S-2045S.
35. Campbell DR, Gross MD, Martini MC, Grandits GA, Slavin JL and Potter JD. Plasma carotenoids as biomarkers of vegetable and fruit intake. Cancer Epidemiol Biomarkers Prev 1994;3:493-500.
36. Carotenoid Database for U.S. Foods. USDA-NCC Carotenoid Database for U.S. Foods - 1998. Internet: http://www.nal.usda.gov/fnic/foodcomp/Data/Carot/ (accessed 1. September 2005).
37. O'Neill ME, Carroll Y, Corridan B, Olmedilla B, Granado F, Blanco I, Van den Berg H, Hininger I, Rousell AM, Chopra M, Southon S, Thurnham DI. A European carotenoid database to assess carotenoid intakes and its use in a five-country comparative study. Br J Nutr. 2001;85:499-507.
38. Ford ES, Gillespie C,Ballew C, Sowell A and Mannino DM. Serum carotenoid concentrations in US children and adolescents. Am J Clin Nutr 2002;76:818-827.

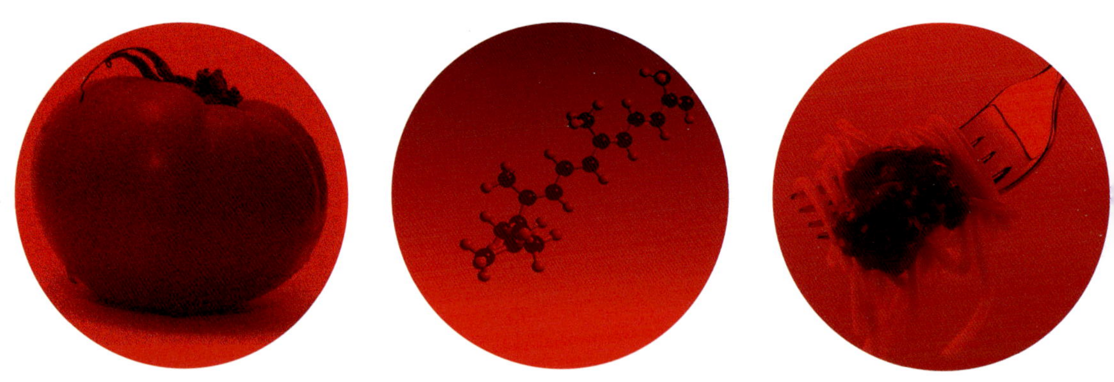

Tomato Lycopene and Bone Health: Preventing Osteoporosis

Dr. L.G. Rao
Calcium Research Laboratory,
Division of Endocrinology & Metabolism
St. Michael s Hospital
Department of Medicine, University of Toronto
Ontario, Canada

Abstract

Lycopene, a potent antioxidant present and primarily found in tomatoes and tomato products, has been associated with human chronic diseases in postmenopausal women based on epidemiological data, clinical studies and *in vitro* cell culture studies. Osteoporosis is a major metabolic bone disease that primarily affects women and men over the age of 50 because of the loss of estrogen at menopause in women and low levels of the sex hormone testosterone in men. One of the risk factors for osteoporosis that is of wide interest and will be reviewed here is oxidative stress caused by reactive oxygen species (ROS). Although oxidative stress has been associated with osteoporosis and the activity and function of osteoblasts and osteoclasts, the two major bone cells involved in the pathogenesis of this disease, the cellular and molecular mechanisms of their actions and the role played by lycopene are not completely clear at the present time. Our ongoing clinical study is the first study to evaluate lycopene from nutritional supplements and tomato juice in the prevention of osteoporosis in postmenopausal women.

INTRODUCTION

There is now convincing evidence of a role for lycopene in osteoporosis. The evidence is based on its potent antioxidant properties, the well-known role of oxidative stress in osteoporosis and the bone cells involved in the pathogenesis of osteoporosis, the studies on the effects of lycopene in these cells in culture and, more recently, the results of a study on lycopene intake and bone resorption markers in postmenopausal women. In order to understand the role of lycopene in osteoporosis, we have included in this review a general discussion on the role of oxidative stress in osteoporosis and bone cells.

OXIDATIVE STRESS AND ANTIOXIDANTS

Reactive oxygen species (ROS) is a collective term which includes superoxide (O_2^-), hydrogen peroxide (H_2O_2), hydroxyl radicals (OH^-) and other free radicals (1,2). ROS are produced from normal metabolic activity and other environmental factors including diet (3). Uncontrolled, ROS will damage different biological targets including lipids, DNA and proteins. ROS production increases with age (4) and is associated with several chronic diseases as illustrated in Figure 1.

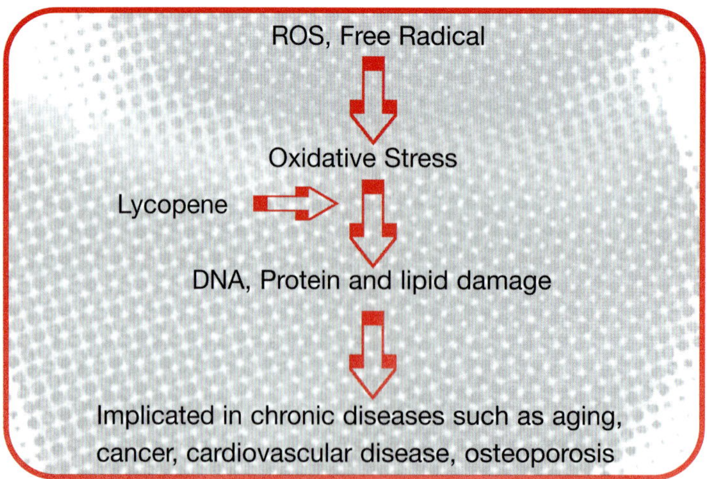

Figure 1: The Role of oxidative stress and the antioxidant lycopene in chronic diseases

Antioxidant defense systems to counteract ROS are present in the body, including superoxide dismutase, glutathione-S peroxidase (GSP), and catalase (5). Additional defense against oxidative stress comes in the form of antioxidants obtained from the diet, notably vitamin C, vitamin E, β-carotene, selenium, lycopene and polyphenols (6). Oxidative stress results from an excess production of ROS (7) and/or the weakening of the antioxidant defense by the body (8) as well as the type of diet(9, 10).

OSTEOPOROSIS IS A MAJOR METABOLIC BONE DISEASE

Bone is a dynamic tissue that is continuously being renewed throughout life by the process of bone remodelling involving the coupled events of the removal of old bone by osteoclasts and the building of new bone by osteoblasts [for review (11, 12)]. The interactions of these cells with multiple molecular agents including hormones, growth factors, and cytokines govern the remodelling process. Metabolic bone diseases, including osteoporosis, result from a disturbance of the bone remodelling process (13, 14). Osteoporosis is a major metabolic bone disease characterized by low bone mass and microarchitectural deterioration of bone tissue, causing enhanced bone fragility and increased risk of fracture (15). Osteoporosis occurs predominantly among women over the age of 50 because of the loss of estrogen at menopause (16) and also among men due to low levels of the sex hormone testosterone (17, 18). It is known as the silent disease that affects one in four women and one in eight men over the age of 50. In postmenopausal bone loss, the remodelling process becomes significantly more active with a primary increase in bone resorption and a counter balancing but insufficient increase in bone formation (19). The early manifestation of the risk of osteoporosis in postmenopausal women is an increase in bone turnover markers of both resorption and formation (16). Bone turnover markers have therefore become measurement parameters to predict risk of fractures among these women (20). Some of the risk factors for osteoporosis are compiled in Table 1 (3,21). The risk factor that will be reviewed in detail here is oxidative stress.

Risk Factors that Can be changed	Risk Factors that Can Not be changed
Low lifetime calcium intake	Genetics
Chronic Inactivity	Race
Excessive Sports Activivty	Sex and Age
Low Body Weight	Previous Fractures
Microgravity	
Hormones	
Medication	
Oxidative stress-related factors Low antioxidant status Smoking Nutrition Deficiency	

Table1: Risk factors for Osteoporosis

ASSOCIATION OF OXIDATIVE STRESS AND ANTIOXIDANTS WITH OSTEOPOROSIS

Oxidative stress has been associated with the pathogenesis of osteoporosis, both in women and men. The severity of osteoporosis was positively correlated with the level of the oxidative stress marker lactic acid in two men with a mitochondrial DNA (mtDNA) deletion (22) and a study of severe osteoporotic syndrome in relatively young males linked osteoporosis to an increase in oxidative stress (23). An increased level of oxidative stress biomarker 8-iso-prostaglandin F alpha (8-iso-PGFα) is biochemically linked with reduced bone density (24, 25). Epidemiological evidence supports the role played by antioxidants in preventing osteoporosis (26,29). Certain antioxidants including vitamin C, E and beta-carotene reduce the risk of osteoporosis and counteract the adverse effects of oxidative stress on bone that are produced during strenuous exercise (28) and by smoking (26).

Vitamins C, E, and A, uric acid, the antioxidant enzymes superoxide dismutase (SOD) and erythrocyte and glutathione peroxidase in plasma were consistently lower in osteoporotic than in control subjects, while plasma levels of malondialdehyde (MDA), the end-product of lipid peroxidation by reactive oxygen species, did not differ between groups. With the exception of unchanged MDA levels, these results showed that antioxidant defenses are markedly decreased in osteoporotic women (30). A negative correlation between SOD and lumbar bone mineral density levels was also found in a study of 31 male patients with primary osteoporosis and 21 subjects as controls (31). A correlation between serum glutathione reductases and bone densitometry values has been reported (32). In spite of these reports, however, the cellular and molecular mechanisms involved in the role of oxidative stress and antioxidants in osteoporosis remain poorly defined.

Low bone density is also associated with oxidative stress in lower species. Thus, melatonin has a bone-protective effect in ovariectomized rats which depends in part on its free radical scavenging properties (33). Ovariectomy, a procedure in rats, which is used to generate models for osteoporosis, induces oxidative stress and impairs the bone antioxidant system in adult rats (34) . A mouse model that has been used to study the role of ROS in age-related disorders including osteoporosis is the accelerated mouse-senescence-prone P/2 (SAM-P/2) that generates increased oxygen radicals (35,36). This model could be very useful in studying the role of lycopene in osteoporosis.

ASSOCIATION OF OXIDATIVE STRESS AND ANTIOXIDANTS WITH OSTEOBLASTS AND OSTEOCLASTS

Osteoclasts, the bone-resorbing cells and osteoblasts, the bone-forming cells, are the two major cells involved in the pathogenesis of osteoporosis. The role of oxidative stress and antioxidants in osteoporosis is mediated through their effects on these cells. A few applicable studies will be reviewed here.

Osteoclasts - The mechanisms involved in the differentiation of osteoclasts and their ability to resorb bone are poorly understood. However, one theory suggests that ROS are involved in this process (37) . Both the H_2O_2 produced by endothelial cells (38) intimately associated with osteoclasts and the H_2O_2 that is produced by osteoclasts (39) increase osteoclastic activity and bone resorption. H_2O_2 may also be involved in the regulation of osteoclast formation , differentiation of osteoclast precursors (41) and osteoclast motility (39). The tartrate-resistant acid phosphatase (TRAP), found on the surface of osteoclasts, has the capacity to react with H_2O_2 to produce highly destructive ROS that target the degradation of collagen and other proteins (42).

Superoxide was localized both intracellularly and at the osteoclast-bone interface using nitroblue tetrazolium (NBT), which is reduced to purple-coloured formazan by ROS, suggesting the participation of superoxide in bone resorption (43), formation and activation of osteoclasts (44). Osteoclastic superoxide is produced by NADPH oxidase (45,46). However, Fraser et al (47) suggested that H_2O_2, but not superoxide, stimulates bone resorption in mouse calvaria and that the earlier finding of stimulation by superoxide (44,48) may be due in part to conversion of this radical to H_2O_2. 1,25-dihydroxyvitamin D_3 ($1,25(OH)_2D_3$) had a direct non-genomic effect on the generation of superoxide anion (O_2^-) which was inhibited by estrogen (49). Estrogen has been reported to have an antioxidant property (50,51). Hormones known to stimulate bone resorption such as parathyroid hormone (PTH) and $1,25(OH)_2D_3$ have stimulatory effects on ROS production in osteoclasts, and hormones known to have inhibitory effect on bone resorption such as calcitonin inhibit ROS production (52,48). The mechanisms involved in the role of oxidative stress in osteoclasts are presently unclear, but a crucial role for ROS in receptor activator of NF-κB ligand (RANKL)-induced osteoclastogenesis has been suggested (53,54).

Antioxidants also play a role in osteoclast activity. Osteoclasts produce the antioxidant enzyme SOD in the plasma membrane (55). ROS production in osteoclasts was inhibited after treating the cells with antioxidant enzymes such as SOD (43) and catalase (40). ROS production in osteoclasts was also inhibited by estrogen (49), the superoxide scavenger deferoxamine mesylate-manganese complex (48,56), pyrrolidine dithiocarbamate (PDTC) and N-acetyl cysteine (NAC) (57). The use of antioxidants from natural sources such as fruits and vegetables could be another way of inhibiting ROS. The use of lycopene in this regard is reviewed below.

Osteoblasts - Very little work has been reported on the role of oxidative stress in osteoblasts. However, previous reports demonstrated that osteoblasts can be induced to produce intracellular ROS (58,59), which can cause a decrease in alkaline phosphatase (ALP) activity and cell death (59); this is partially inhibited by vitamin E (58). Treatment of rat osteosarcoma ROS 17/2.8 cells with tumour necrosis factor-alpha (TNF-α) suppressed bone sialoprotein (BSP) gene transcription through a tyrosine kinase-dependent pathway that generates ROS (60). H_2O_2 modulated intracellular calcium (Ca^{2+}) activity in osteoblasts by increasing Ca^{2+} release from the intracellular Ca^{2+} stores (61). Oxidative stress induced by a variety of compounds such as xanthine/xanthine oxidase (XXO) and minimally oxidized LDL (MO-LDL) has been shown to inhibit the osteogenic differentiation of osteoprogenitor cells (62). The mechanisms involved in the role played by ROS in osteoblasts are not clear, but a suggestion has been proposed that ROS stimulates RANKL expression via extracellular signal-regulated kinases (ERKs) and the protein kinase-cAMP response element-binding protein (PKA-CREB) pathway in mouse osteoblasts and via ERKs and heat shock factor 2 (HSF2) in human MG63 cells (63).

THE POTENT ANTIOXIDANT LYCOPENE

The chemistry of lycopene and its potent antioxidant properties have been reviewed in other chapters of this book. Only the studies of lycopene in bone cells and clinical studies in postmenopausal women at risk of osteoporosis will be reviewed here.

IN VITRO STUDIES OF LYCOPENE IN BONE CELLS

Effects of lycopene on osteoclasts - To date, there are only two reported studies on the effects of lycopene in osteoclasts (64,65) . Rao et al (65) cultured cells from bone marrow prepared from rat femur in 16-well calcium phosphate-coated Osteologic™ multi-test slides (Millenium Biologix Inc).

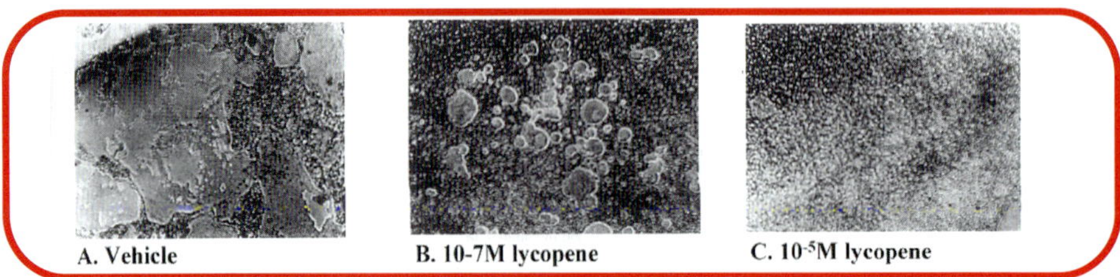

Figure 2: Photomicrograph showing the effect of lycopene on resorption of the calcium phosphate substrate coating of Osteologic Multi-test Slides™. Vehicle or lycopene was added on the day of plating and at every medium change thereafter. At day 8, the cells were removed with sodium hypochlorite and the resorption pit photographed under the microscope. (Magnification, x 40. (Rao LG et al, 2003).

Varying concentrations of lycopene in the absence or presence of the resorbing agent PTH-(1-34) were added at the start of culture and at each medium change every 48 hours. The effects of lycopene on mineral resorption is shown in Figure 2. Lycopene inhibition of the TRAP+ multinucleated osteoclasts formation and NBT-staining were studied. Lycopene inhibited the TRAP+ multinucleated cell formation in both vehicle- and PTH-treated cultures (Figure 3).

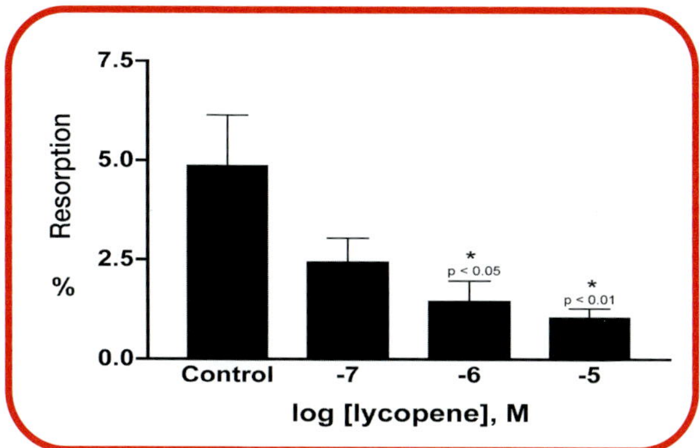

Figure 3: Effect of lycopene on PTH-stimulated osteoclastic bone resorption. Vehicle or lycopene was added on the day of plating and at every medium change thereafter. At day 8, the cells were removed with sodium hypochlorite and the resorption pit analyzed using the Microst Reader. The bars represent mean ± SEM of 16 determinations from four experiments. *, P <0 .01; **, P<0 .05. (Rao LG, 2003)

The cells that were stained with the NBT reduction product formazan were decreased by treatment with 10^{-5} M lycopene (Figure 4) indicating that lycopene inhibited the formation of ROS-secreting osteoclasts. Rao et al concluded that lycopene inhibited basal and PTH-stimulated osteoclastic mineral resorption and formation of TRAP+ multinucleated osteoclasts, as well as the ROS produced by osteoclasts. These findings are new and may be important in the pathogenesis, treatment and prevention of osteoporosis.

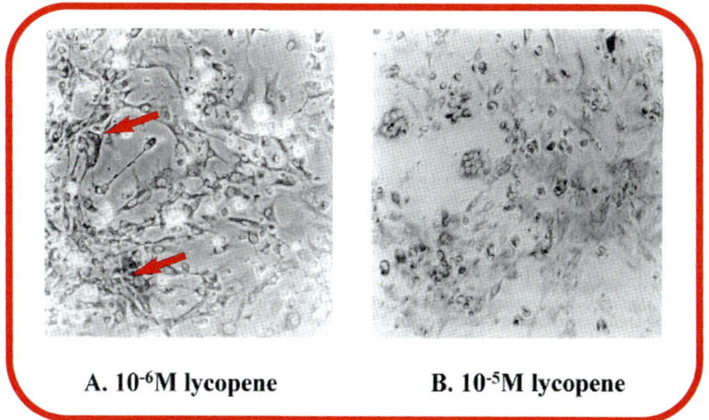

Figure 4: Effect of lycopene on Reactive Oxygen Species (ROS) production in osteoclasts. Stains in panel A (arrows) represent ROS production by osteoclasts. (Magnification, x 40) (Rao LG et al, 2003)

The effects of lycopene on osteoclast formation and bone resorption were also reported by Ishimi et al using murine osteoclasts formed in co-culture with calvarial osteoblasts (64). Their results differed from those of Rao et al (65) in that they found that lycopene inhibited the PTH-induced, but not the basal, TRAP+ multinucleated cell formation. Furthermore, they could not demonstrate any effect of lycopene on bone resorption. They also did not study the effect of lycopene on ROS production.

Effects of lycopene on osteoblasts – The studies on the effects of lycopene on osteoblasts are limited to two reports (66,67). Kim et al (67) showed that lycopene stimulated the proliferation of the osteoblast-like SaOS-2 cells as shown in Figure 5.

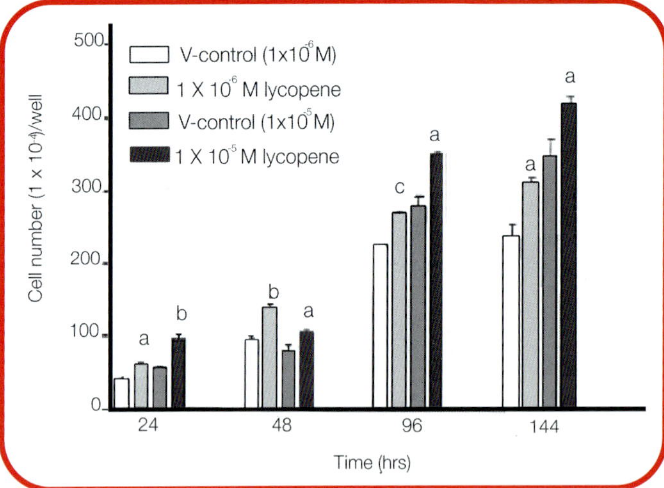

Figure 5: Time course of the stimulatory effect of lycopene on the proliferation of SaOS-2 cells. After 24 hours in culture, SaOS-2 cells were treated with various concentrations of lycopene and further incubated for the time periods specified in the figure. Compared with respective vehicle control of the same dilution, a = P <0.05; b = P<0.001; c = P<0.005. (Kim L et al, 2003)

They also reported that lycopene had a stimulatory effect on ALP activity, a marker of osteoblastic differentiation in more mature cells but, depending on the time of addition, had an inhibitory or no effect on younger SaOS-Dex cells (Figure 6).

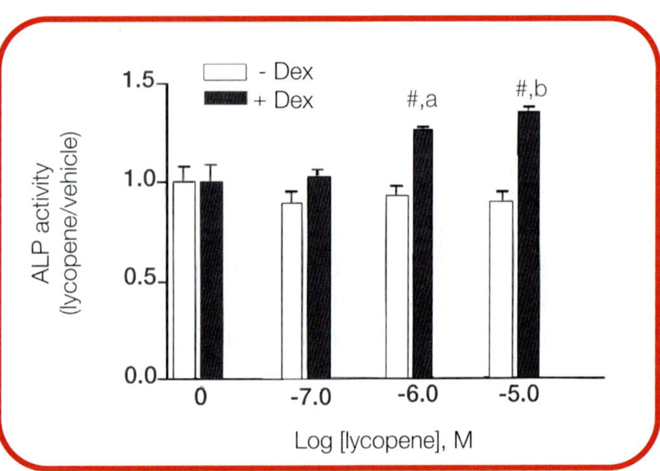

Figure 6: Effect on ALP activity of lycopene added at day 6 of culture in the presence (SaOS+Dex) or absence (SaOS-Dex) of Dex, with further incubation for 24 hours. Comparisons between SaOS-Dex cells and SaOS+Dex cells at the same dilution were as follows: # = P < .005; & = P < .005. Comparisons with zero control were as follows: a = P< .05; b = P < .01. (Kim L et al, 2003).

These findings were the first report on the effect of lycopene on human osteoblasts. In another study by Park et al (66), the effect of lycopene on MC3T3 cells (the mouse osteoblastic cells) was contrary to the findings of Kim et al (67). Park demonstrated that lycopene had an inhibitory effect on cell proliferation. Both studies, however, reported that ALP activity was stimulated. The discrepancy in the effect of lycopene on cell proliferation could be a result of species differences or experimental conditions. More studies are required to clarify the role of lycopene in osteoblasts.

CLINICAL STUDIES ON THE ROLE OF LYCOPENE IN POSTMENOPAUSAL WOMEN AT RISK OF OSTEOPOROSIS

Postmenopause is associated with a global increase in bone turnover markers (68,69) that predict bone loss and osteoporosis in postmenopausal women (19). One of the objectives of our current clinical study at St. Michael's Hospital is to test whether the serum lycopene correlates inversely with the oxidative stress parameters and bone turnover markers in postmenopausal women who are at risk of osteoporosis. Thirty-three women aged 50-60 were recruited and asked to complete a seven-day food intake record prior to giving fasting blood samples. Oxidative stress parameters, total antioxidant capacity, serum lycopene and the bone turnover markers ALP (bone formation) and cross-linked N-telopeptides of type I collagen (NTx) (bone resorption) were measured from serum samples. The participants were grouped into quartiles according to their serum lycopene per kilogram body weight (nM/kg) and correlation analyses were carried out using the Newman-Keuls post test. The most important and interesting findings to date are the significant decreases in protein oxidation as indicated by increased thiols ($p<0.05$) and decreased NTx values ($p<0.005$) as levels of serum lycopene increase (Figure 7) (70).

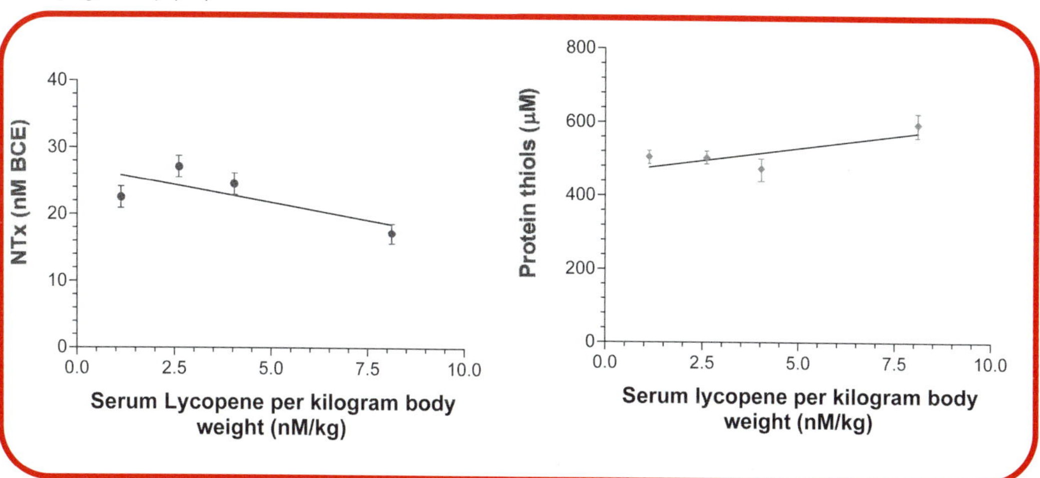

Since there was a significant positive correlation between serum lycopene levels and dietary lycopene intake as determined from the estimated food records ($p<0.01$) (Figure 8), our results support the hypothesis that dietary lycopene acts as an effective antioxidant, reducing oxidative stress and bone turnover markers. Our observations suggest an important role for lycopene mediated via its antioxidant property in reducing the risk of osteoporosis. Dietary intervention studies with varying doses and sources of lycopene are currently being conducted to determine the beneficial effects of lycopene in the prevention and management of osteoporosis.

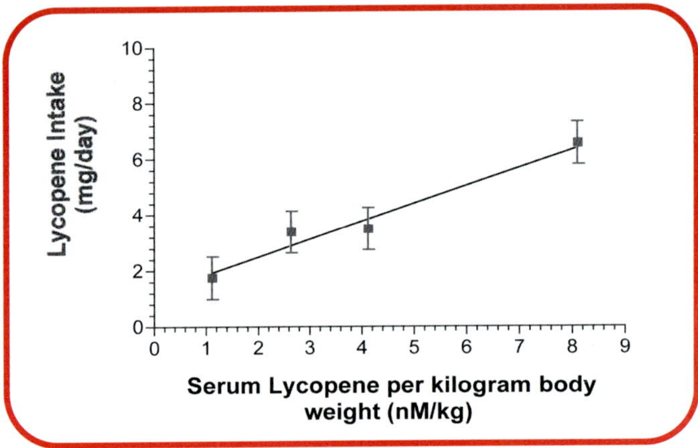

Figure 8: Effect of lycopene intake on serum lycopene in 33 postmenopausal women participants. (Rao LG et al, 2005)

CONCLUSION

Although there is epidemiological evidence to support the beneficial effects of tomatoes and tomato products in the prevention of osteoporosis in the Mediterranean population, the direct role of lycopene, the potent antioxidant component in tomatoes, has not yet been explored. The effects of lycopene on osteoblasts (66,67) and osteoclasts (64,65) that have been reported and the involvement of oxidative stress in the pathogenesis of osteoporosis reviewed above provide evidence for the importance of lycopene in the prevention of osteoporosis. Our ongoing clinical study is the first study to evaluate lycopene in the prevention of osteoporosis in postmenopausal women. Although it is too early to suggest that eating tomatoes and tomato products will prevent osteoporosis, it would be a healthy practice to include tomatoes and tomato products in the diet as a source of lycopene for the prevention of oxidative stress-related chronic diseases, including osteoporosis. The final results of our study may indicate that lycopene can be used either as a dietary alternative to drug therapy or as a complement to the drugs used by women at risk for osteoporosis.

REFERENCES:

1. Sahnoun Z, Jamoussi K, Zeghal KM. Free radicals and antioxidants: human physiology, pathology and therapeutic aspects. Therapie 1997;52:251-570.
2. Halliwell B. Free radicals, antioxidants and human disease: curiosity, cause or consequence? Lancet 1994;344:721-4.
3. Rao LG, Gunns M, Rao AV. The role of lycopene in the prevention of chronic diseases. Agro Food Industry Hi Tech. 2003;1:25-30.
4. Schoneich C. Reactive oxygen species and biological aging: a mechanistic approach. Experimental Gerontology 1999;34:19-34.
5. Knight JA. The biochemistry of aging. [Review] [289 refs]. Advances in Clinical Chemistry. 2000;35:1-62.
6. Giovannucci E. Tomatoes, tomato-based products, lycopene, and cancer: review of the epidemiologic literature. J National Cancer Institute 1999;91:317-31.
7. Galli F, Piroddi M, Annetti C, Aisa C, Floridi E, Floridi A. Oxidative stress and reactive oxygen species. Contributions to Nephrology 2005;149:240-60.
8. Jacob RA, Burri BJ. Oxidative damage and defense. American Journal of Clinical Nutrition 1996;63:985S-90S.
9. Smolkova B, Dusinska M, Raslova K, McNeill G, Spustova V, Blazicek P, et al. Seasonal changes in markers of oxidative damage to lipids and DNA; correlations with seasonal variation in diet. Mutation Research 2004;551:135-44.
10. Farombi EO, Hansen M, Ravn-Haren G, Moller P, Dragsted LO. Commonly consumed and naturally occurring dietary substances affect biomarkers of oxidative stress and DNA damage in healthy rats. Food & Chemical Toxicology 2004;42:1315-22.
11. Chan GK, Duque G. Age-related bone loss: old bone, new facts. Gerontology 2002;48:62-71.
12. Mundy GR. Bone Remodeling. In MJ F, editor. Primer on the Metabolic Bone Diseases and Disorders of Mineral Metabolism. New York: Lippincott Williams & Wilkins; 1999. p. 30-8.
13. Raisz LG. Bone cell biology: new approaches and unanswered questions. J Bone Min Res 1993;8:S457-S65.
14. Lindsay R, Cosman F. Prevention of Osteoporosis. In Favus MJ, editor. Primer on the Metabolic Bone Diseases and Disorders of Mineral Metabolism. New York: Lippincott Williams & Wilkins; 1999. p. 264-70.
15. Consensus Development Conference. Diagnosis, prophylaxis and treatment of osteoporosis. American Journal of Medicine 1993;94:646-50.
16. Raisz LG. Pathogenesis of osteoporosis: concepts, conflicts, and prospects. Journal of Clinical Investigation 2005;115:3318-25.
17. Amin S. Male osteoporosis: epidemiology and pathophysiology. [Review]. Current Osteoporosis Reports 2003;1:71-7.
18. Pietschmann P, Kerschan-Schindl K. Osteoporosis: gender-specific aspects. Wiener Medizinische Wochenschrift 2004;154:411-5.
19. Garnero P, Sornay-Rendu E, Chapuy M-C, Delmas PD. Increased bone turnover in late posmenopausal women is a major determinant of osteoporosis. J Bon Min Res 1996;11:337-49.
20. Srivastava AK, Vliet EL, Lewiecki EM, Maricic M, Abdelmalek A, Gluck O, et al. Clinical use of serum and urine bone markers in the management of osteoporosis. Current Medical Research & Opinion. 2005;21:1015-26.

21. Bartl R, Frisch B. Chapter 5 Recognizing Risk Factors. In Osteoporosis: Diagnosis, prevention, therapy. New York: Springer-Verlag; 2004. p. 40-8.
22. Varanasi SS, Francis RM, Berger CE, Papiha SS, Datta HK. Mitochondrial DNA deletion associated oxidative stress and severe male osteoporosis. Osteoporosis International. 1999;10:143-9.
23. Polidori MC, Stahl W, Eichler O, Niestroj I, Sies H. Profiles of antioxidants in human plasma. Free Rad Biol Med 2001;30:456-62.
24. Basu S, Michaelsson K, Olofsson H, Johansson S, Melhus H. Association between oxidative stress and bone mineral density. Biochemical & Biophysical Research Communications 2001;288:275-9.
25. Sontakke AN, Tare RS. A duality in the roles of reactive oxygen species with respect to bone metabolism. Clinica Chimica Acta 2002;318:145-8.
26. Melhus H, Michaelsson K, Holmberg L, Wolk A, Ljunghall S. Smoking, antioxidant vitamins, and the risk of hip fracture. Journal of Bone & Mineral Research 1999;14:129-35.
27. Morton DJ, Barrett-Connor EL, Schneider DL. Vitamin C supplement and bone mineral density in postmenopausal women. J Bon Min Res 2001;16:135-40.
28. Singh VN. A current perspective on nutrition and exercise. J Nutr 1992;122:760-5.
29. Leveille SG, LaCroix AZ, Koepsell TD, Beresford SA, VanBelle G, Buchner DM. Dietary vitamin C and bone mineral density in postmenopausal women in Washington State, USA. J Epidemiol Community Health 1997;51:479-85.
30. Maggio D, Barabani M, Pierandrei M, Polidori MC, Catani M, Mecocci P, et al. Marked decrease in plasma antioxidants in aged osteoporotic women: results of a cross-sectional study. Journal of Clinical Endocrinology & Metabolism 2003;88:1523-7.
31. Yalin S, Bagis S, Polat G, Dogruer N, Cenk Aksit S, Hatungil R, et al. Is there a role of free oxygen radicals in primary male osteoporosis?. Clinical & Experimental Rheumatology 2005;23:689-92.
32. Avitabile M, Campagna NE, Magri GA, Vinci M, Sciacca G, Alia G, et al. Correlation between serum glutathione reductases and bone densitometry values]. [Italian]. Bollettino - Societa Italiana Biologia Sperimentale 1991;67:931-7.
33. Cardinali DP, Ladizesky MG, Boggio V, Cutrera RA, Mautalen C. Melatonin effects on bone: experimental facts and clinical perspectives. Journal of Pineal Research. 34(2):81-7, 2003 March. 2003;34:81-7.
34. Muthusami S, Ramachandran I, Muthusamy B, Vasudevan G, Prabhu V, Subramaniam V, et al. Ovariectomy induces oxidative stress and impairs bone antioxidant system in adult rats. Clinica Chimica Acta 2005;360:81-6.
35. Udagawa N. Mechanisms involved in bone resorption. Biogerontology 2002;3:79-83.
36. Hosokawa M. A higher oxidative status accelerates senescence and aggravates age-dependent disorders in SAMP strains of mice. Mechanisms of Ageing & Development 2002;123:1553-61.
37. Silverton S. Osteoclast radicals. Journal of Cellular Biochemistry. 1994;56:367-73.
38. Zaidi M, Alam AS, Bax BE, Shankar VS, Bax CM, Gill JS, et al. Role of the endothelial cell in osteoclast control: new perspectives. Bone 1993;14:97-102.
39. Bax BE, Alam AS, Banerji B, Bax CM, Bevis PJ, Stevens CR, et al. Stimulation of osteoclastic bone resorption by hydrogen peroxide. Biochemical & Biophysical Research Communications 1992;183:1153-8.
40. Suda N, Morita I, Kuroda T, Murota S. Participation of oxidative stress in the process of osteoclast differentiation. Biochimica et Biophysica Acta 1993;1157:318-23.

41. Steinbeck MJ, Kim JK, Trudeau MJ, Hauschka PV, Karnovsky MJ. Involvement of hydrogen peroxide in the differentiation of clonal HD-11EM cells into osteoclast-like cells. Journal of Cellular Physiology 1998;176:574-87.
42. Halleen JM, Raisanen S, Salo JJ, Reddy SV, Roodman GD, Hentunen TA, et al. Intracellular fragmentation of bone resorption products by reactive oxygen species generated by osteoclastic tartrate-resistant acid phosphatase. Journal of Biological Chemistry 1999;274:22907-10.
43. Key LL, Ries WL, Taylor RG, Hays BD, Pitzer BL. Oxygen derived free radicals in osteoclasts: the specificity and location of the nitroblue tetrazolium reaction. Bone 1990;11:115-9.
44. Garrett IR, Boyce BF, Oreffo ROC, Bonewald L, Pser J, Mundy GR. Oxygen-derived free radicals stimulate osteoclastic bone resorption in rodent bone in vitro and in vivo. J Clin Invest 1990;85:632-9.
45. Darden AG, Ries WL WW, Rodriguiz RM, Key Jr LL. Osteoclastic superoxide production and bone resorption: stimulation and inhibition by modulators ofn NADPH oxidase. J Bon Min Res 1996;11:671-5.
46. Steinbeck MJ, Appel WH Jr., Verhoeven AJ, Karnovsky MJ. NADPH-oxidase expression and in situ production of superoxide by osteoclasts actively resorbing bone. Journal of Cell Biology;126:765-72.
47. Fraser JH, Helfrich MH, Wallace HM, Ralston SH. Hydrogen peroxide, but not superoxide, stimulates bone resorption in mouse calvariae. Bone 1996;19:223-6.
48. Key LL, Wolf WC, Gundberg CM, Ries WL. Superoxide and bone resorption. Bone 1994;15:431-6.
49. Berger CE, Horrocks BR, Datta HK. Direct non-genomic effect of steroid hormones on superoxide generation in the bone resorbing osteoclasts. Molecular and Cellular Endocrinology 1999;149:53-9.
50. Wagner AH, Schroeter MR, Hecker M. 17b-estradiol inhibition of NADPH oxidase expression in human endothelial cells. FASEB J 2001;15:2121-30.
51. Clarke R, Leonessa F, Welch JN, Skaar TC. Cellular and molecular pharmacology of antiestrogen action and resistance. Pharmacol Rev 2001;53:25-71.
52. Datta HK, Rathod H, Manning P, Turnbull Y, McNeil CJ. Parathyroid hormone induces superoxide anion burst in the osteoclasts: evidence of the direct instantaneous activation of the osteoclast by the hormone. J Endocrinology 1996;149:269-75.
53. Ha H, Kwak HB, Lee SW, Jin HM, Kim HM, Kim HH, et al. Reactive oxygen species mediate RANK signaling in osteoclasts. Experimental Cell Research 2004;301:119-27.
54. Lee NK, Choi YG, Baik JY, Han SY, Jeong DW, Bae YS, et al. A crucial role for reactive oxygen species in RANKL-induced osteoclast differentiation. Blood 2005;106:852-9.
55. Oursler MJ, Collin-Osdoby P, Li L, Schmitt E, Osdoby P. Evidence for an immunological and functional relationship between superoxide dismutase and a high molecular weight osteoclast plasma membrane glycoprotein. Journal of Cellular Biochemistry 1991;46:331-44.
56. Ries WL, Key LL, Rodriguiz RM. Nitroblue tetrazolium reduction and bone resorption by osteoclasts in vitro inhibited by a manganese-based superoxide dismutase mimic. J Bone Min Res 1992;1992:931-8.
57. Hall TJ, SchaeublinM, Fuller K, Chambers TJ. The role of oxygen intermediates in osteoclastic bone resorption. Biochem. Biophys. Res. Commun. 1995;207:280-7.

58. Cortizo AM, Bruzzone L, Molinuevo S, Etcheverry SB. A possible role of oxidative stress in the vanadium-induced cytotoxicity in the MC3T3E1 osteoblast and UMR106 osteosarcoma cell lines. Toxicology 2000;147:89-99.
59. Liu H-C, Cheng R-M, Lin F-H, Fang H-W. Sintered beta-dicalcium phosphate particles induce intracellular reactive oxygen species in rat osteoblasts. Biomed Eng Appl Basis Commun 1999;11:259-64.
60. Samoto H, Shimizu E, Matsuda-Honjo Y, Saito R, Yamazaki M, Kasai K, et al. TNF-alpha suppresses bone sialoprotein (BSP) expression in ROS17/2.8 cells. Journal of Cellular Biochemistry 2002;87:313-23.
61. Nam SH, Jung SY, Yoo CM, Ahn EH, Suh CK. H_2O_2 enhances Ca^{2+} release from osteoblast internal stores. Yonsei Medical Journal 2002;43:229-35.
62. Shouhed D, Kha HT, Richardson JA, Amantea CM, Hahn TJ, Parhami F. Osteogenic oxysterols inhibit the adverse effects of oxidative stress on osteogenic differentiation of marrow stromal cells. Journal of Cellular Biochemistry 2005;95:1276-83.
63. Bai XC, Lu D, Liu AL, Zhang ZM, Li XM, Zou ZP, et al. Reactive oxygen species stimulates receptor activator of NF-kappaB ligand expression in osteoblast. Journal of Biological Chemistry 2005;280:17497-506.
64. Ishimi Y, Ohmura M, Wang X, Yamaguchi M, Ikegami S. Inhibition by carotenoids and retinoic acid of osteoclast-like cell formation induced by bone-resorbing agents in vitro. J Clin Biochem Nutr 1999;27:113-22.
65. Rao LG, Krishnadev N, Banasikowska K, Rao AV. Lycopene I - Effect on osteoclasts: Lycopene inhibits basal and parathyroid hormone-stimulated osteoclast formation and mineral resorption mediated by reactive oxygen species in rat bone marrow cultures. J Med Food 2003;6:69-78.
66. Park CK, Ishimi Y, Ohmura M, Yamaguchi M, Ikegami S. Vitamin A and carotenoids stimulate differentiation of mouse osteoblastic cells. J Nutr Sci Vitaminol 1997; 43:281-96.
67. Kim L, Rao AV, Rao LG. Lycopene II - Effect on osteoblasts: The caroteroid lycopene stimulates cell proliferation and alkaline phosphatase activity of SaOS-2 cells. J Med Food 2003;6:79-86.
68. Vernejoul M-C de. Markers of bone remodelling in metabolic bone disease. Drugs & Aging 1998;1 (suppl1):9-14.
69. Kushida K, Takahashi M, Kawana K, Inoue T. Comparison of markers for bone formation and resorption in premenopausal and postmenopausal subjects, and osteoporosis patients. J Clin Endocr Metab. 1995;80:2447-50.
70. Rao LG, Collins ES, Josse RG, Strauss A, Rao AV. Lycopene consumption significantly decreases oxidative stress and bone resorption markers in postmenopausal women at risk for osteoporosis. Joint Meeting of the ECTS and IBMS 2005; June 25-29, Geneva, Switzerland.

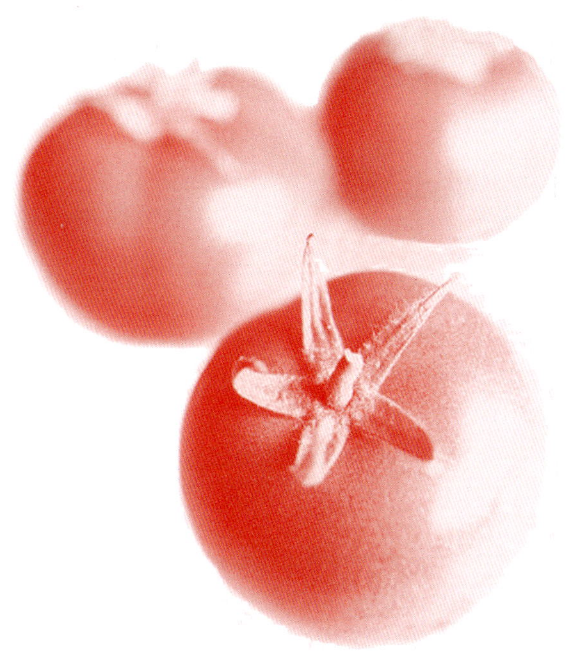

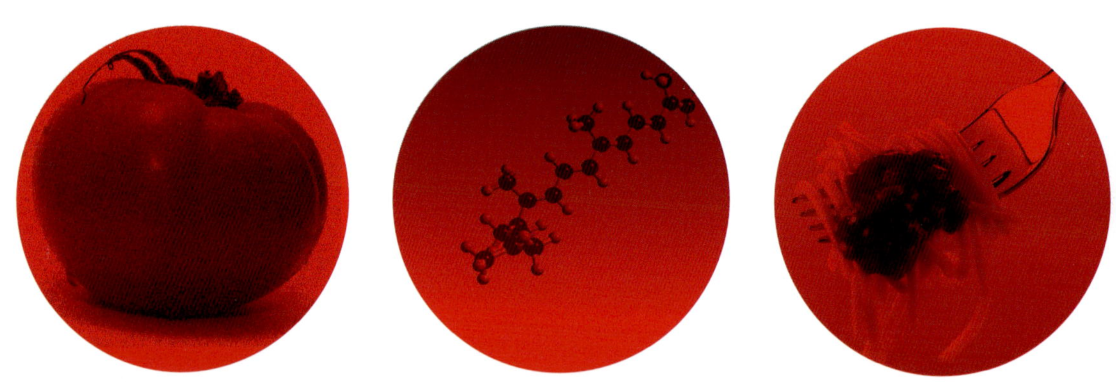

Reducing Hypertension with Tomato Lycopene

Dr.Esther Paran
Hypertension Unit,
Soroka University Medical Centre,
Faculty of Health Sciences,
Ben Gurion University of the Negev,
Beer Sheba, Israel

Abstract

Hypertension is considered the most common risk factor for cardio and cerebrovascular target organ damage and renal disease. Normalization of blood pressure with antihypertensive therapy has a beneficial effect; with stroke incidence reduced by 40 to 50 percent, MI by 20 percent and congestive heart failure by more than 50 percent. Lifestyle modification by dietary changes can reduce BP. Therefore according to guidelines, all patients should undergo appropriate lifestyle modification as the first step of their treatment.

In recent years, reactive oxidative species (ROS) have been suggested as playing a major role in the pathogenesis of hypertension. Oxidative stress is associated with atherosclerosis and hypertension. Vascular oxidative stress has been demonstrated in experimental hypertensive animal models and clinical hypertension. Dietary supplementation of fruits and vegetables has been linked to a rise in plasma vitamin antioxidant levels and to reduction in blood pressure values. In the NHANES III study, a one-SD higher level in β-carotene was associated with an 11% lower risk of hypertension, and the serum β–carotene level was inversely related to systolic blood pressure (SBP). Tomato extract contains carotenoids such as lycopene, β-carotene and vitamin E which are known to be effective antioxidants, can inactivate free radicals, and have been shown to slow progression of atherosclerosis. In the Kuopio Ischaemic Heart Disease Risk Factor

study a low serum lycopene concentration was found to be associated with a higher intima-media thickness. As increased thickness of the intima-media has been shown to predict coronary events and stroke, lycopene intakes and serum concentrations may have clinical and public health relevance.
In spite of these promising findings, prospective randomized studies evaluating the effect of different antioxidant vitamins on blood pressure levels are spare.
We evaluated the effect of tomato extract on systolic and diastolic blood pressure in grade 1 HT in two different studies. In the first trial untreated mild hypertensive patients received tomato extract for 8 weeks in a double blind placebo controlled study. Systolic and diastolic blood pressure decreased significantly together with a drop in oxidative stress markers.
The second study was designed to evaluate the change in systolic and diastolic blood pressure among treated but uncontrolled hypertensives following treatment with tomato extract. Fifty-four moderate but inadequately controlled hypertensive subjects, without concomitant diseases were randomized and after a routine baseline evaluation, the study participants entered two double blind cross-over treatment periods of 6 weeks each, with standardized tomato extract or identical placebo. Daily oral supplementation of tomato extract * significantly decreased SBP and DBP in treated but uncontrolled hypertensives, concordantly with increase in serum lycopene and nitrate levels. Therefore we attribute the reduction in blood pressure to antioxidant activity of the tomato extract and increase in NO.
Conclusions: A short term treatment with antioxidant-rich tomato extract can reduce blood pressure in mild to moderate hypertensives. The positive results of these trials are encouraging. However, the studies are relatively small and the treatment periods were short. The continuous effect of this treatment and the long term beneficial effect on cardiovascular risk factors still need to be demonstrated.

Key words: Hypertension, oxidative stress, antioxidants, tomato extract, lycopene, carotenoids.

INTRODUCTION

Hypertension is the most common reason for office visits of adults to physicians in the United States and for use of prescription drugs. According to recent data the incidence of hypertension in the 18 years and older population of the United States is approximately 30 percent (1,2). The number of patients with hypertension is likely

*(Lyc-O-Mato®)

to grow as the population ages, since either isolated systolic hypertension or combined systolic and diastolic hypertension occurs in over one half of the persons older than 65 years. Hypertension is considered the most common risk factor for cardio and cerebrovascular target organ damage such as heart attack, congestive heart failure and ischemic and hemorrhagic stroke (3,4). The likelihood of developing these complications varies with the severity of hypertension. Normalization of blood pressure [BP] with antihypertensive therapy has beneficial effect; stroke incidence reduced by 40 to 50 percent, MI by 20 percent and congestive heart failure by more than 50 percent.

According to the latest guidelines: the JNC VII (5) and recommendations of the ESH (6), the increase in risk starts already with blood pressure above 110/75 mmHg (7,8) and is farther increased by the presence of risk factors (9). According to these guidelines, all patients should undergo appropriate lifestyle modification as the first step of their treatment. In the mild cases, such as high normal or "prehypertensive" patients (systolic BP between130-139 mmHg and or diastolic BP between 85-89 mmHg), and grade I hypertensives (systolic BP between140-159 mmHg and /or diastolic BP between 90-99 mmHg), nonpharmacologic therapy will be the only treatment for the first 6 to 12 months.

For primary prevention of hypertension the 2002 recommendations of The National High Blood Pressure Education Program Coordinating Committee involve a population-based approach and an intensive targeted strategy focused on individuals at high risk for hypertension. The very recent publication of the AHA Scientific Statement includes detailed recommendation for the non-pharmacologic, mostly dietetic approach to mild hypertension, prehypertension and high normal individuals. They emphasize that the well-established dietary modifications that lower BP are reduced salt intake, weight loss, and moderation of alcohol consumption (among those who drink). In non-hypertensive individuals, dietary changes can lower BP and prevent hypertension. In uncomplicated stage I hypertension (SBP of 140 to 159 mmHg or DBP of 90 to 99 mmHg), dietary changes serve as initial treatment before drug therapy (10).
The sixth edition of *Dietary Guidelines for Americans*, issued by the Departments of Health and Human Services (HHS) and Agriculture (USDA), recommends reduced calorie consumption, increased physical activity and wiser food choices. For an average 2,000-calorie intake, 2 cups of fruit and 2½ cups of vegetables per day are recommended (USDA Jan 2006). These guidelines, and many others around the world, are based on the large body of publication and experience with the DASH diet (Dietary Approaches to Stop Hypertension), which is rich in fruits, vegetables, and low-fat dairy foods and significantly lowers blood pressure (11).
Several mechanisms have been proposed for this dietary effect on BP, including an

increased vitamin and nutrient intake of antioxidant compounds. However, interventional trials of vitamin supplements to elevate circulating plasma concentrations of antioxidant vitamins have produced little evidence to support this hypothesis (12,13).

Current evidence therefore points to the beneficial effects of eating more fruit and vegetables rather than vitamin supplementation (14).

OXIDATIVE STRESS AND HYPERTENSION

In recent years, reactive oxidative species (ROS) have been suggested as playing a major role in the pathogenesis of hypertension. Oxidative stress is associated with several other cardiovascular diseases, including atherosclerosis, heart failure, stroke and diabetes (15). Physiologically vascular ROS is produced in all layers of the vessel wall in a controlled manner. Under pathological conditions, as hypertension, the increased concentration of superoxide ($O_2^{\bullet}$) inactivates nitric oxide (NO). The loss of bioactivity of NO in the vessel wall is the main reason for impaired endothelial function. This endothelial damage may account for the increased peripheral resistance, a characteristic finding of chronic essential hypertension (16,17).

The dominant role for NAD(P)H oxidase in production of vascular ROS is evident from the marked up-regulation of its level in most of the cardiovascular diseases. Superoxides are the main precursors of ROS in the vasculature, while NAD(P)H oxidase is its primary source. Superoxide anions and other free radicals decrease the availability of NO by reacting with NO, resulting in attenuated intrinsic vasodilating activity (18).

Vascular oxidative stress has been demonstrated in spontaneous and experimental hypertensive animal models. Spontaneously hypertensive rats (SHR) exhibit increased NAD(P)H driven $O_2^{\bullet}$ generation in resistance vessels. This is associated with NAD(P)H oxidase subunit over expression and enhanced oxidase activity (19,20).

Superoxide is increased in the kidney of SHR as well and in other different experimental hypertension animal models (21).

Clinical studies demonstrated increased ROS production in patients with essential hypertension (22,23). These findings are based, in general, on increased levels of plasma thiobarbituric acid reactive substances and 8-epi-isoprostanes, biomarkers of lipid peroxidation and oxidative stress.

Redon et al evaluated the oxidative status in whole blood and mononuclear peripherals cells and their relationship with blood pressure in human hypertension (24). In both, whole blood and peripheral mononuclear cells oxidized/reduced glutathione ratio and malondialdehyde was significantly higher, and the activity of superoxide dismutase, catalase, and glutathione peroxidase was significantly lower in hypertensive patients when compared with normal subjects. The content of damaged base 8-oxo-2'-deoxyguanosine in nuclear and mitochondrial deoxyribonucleoproteins of hypertensive subjects was also significantly higher than that of the normotensive control subjects. Their conclusions were that in hypertensive subjects, oxidative stress is increased and the activity of antioxidant mechanisms is reduced in a way apparently independent of the blood pressure values.

Activation of the renin-angiotensin system [RAS] has been shown to be involved in increased ROS production in several studies. Chronic infusion of angiotensin II (Ang II) even in non pressure concentrations increases BP after a few days. This increased hypertensive response is accompanied by oxidative stress as measured by plasma isoprostanes (25). Moreover, isoprostanes and superoxide anions can exert a direct vasoconstrictor effect (26). Ang II also increased vascular production of superoxide anion via an NAD(P)H oxidase (27). Ang II is shown to induce a dose-dependent activation of NADPH oxidase in human neutrophils and monocytes (28).

ANTIOXIDANTS AND HYPERTENSION

Under physiologic conditions, endogenous antioxidants bolster defenses to minimize the interaction between $O_2^{\bullet}$ and NO. This tenuous balance seems to be altered in a variety of common disease states. These include hypertension, diabetes, cigarette smoking and heart failure (29). In animal models and in human diseases with enhanced degradation of NO by ROS, antioxidant vitamins have been shown to enhance endothelium-dependent vasodilation, indicating improved endothelial function (30,16,31). However, reduction of blood pressure itself does not restore endothelial function and does not decrease oxidative stress components. Some treatments used to lower BP, such as RAS antagonists: angiotensin converting enzyme [ACE] inhibitors or Ang II receptor blockers, can restore endothelium-dependent relaxation response to acetylcholine and improve inflammatory parameters in the vessel wall (32). It seems that the RAS antagonists, by reducing the production of Ang II, improve the balance between pro- and anti-oxidant substances in the endothelium of arterioles.

DIETARY INTERVENTIONS AND BLOOD PRESSURE

Several observational epidemiological studies and a few clinical trials have suggested an inverse association between dietary intake of fruits and vegetables and BP. These trials have been based mainly on change of the whole dietary pattern as the DASH diet or the Oxford Fruit and Vegetable Study Group (33,14,34). However, studies conducted with the edition of vitamins or nutritional substances revealed conflicting results. Several studies have shown an inverse association between serum levels of vitamin C and BP, and the same has been shown for vitamin E and β–carotene (35,36).

The NHANES III trial, has examined the cross-sectional relationship between the serum β–carotene level and BP. In that study, a one-SD higher level in β–carotene was associated with an 11% lower risk of hypertension, and the serum β–carotene level was inversely related to SBP (37).

Several small, short-term clinical trials testing high doses of vitamin C on BP have been inconsistent (38-40), and a 5 year randomized trial was not able to demonstrate any effect on BP (41). The potential value of the antioxidants vitamin E, β–carotene and vitamin C for secondary prevention has been evaluated in a number of clinical trials with largely no benefit. This included a lack of benefit from vitamin E in the HOPE trial (13) and from combined therapy in the Heart Protection Study (42).

A recent study assessed the effects of supplementation of antioxidant vitamins and trace elements, at nutritional doses, (SU.VI.MAX. trial) on the risk of hypertension over a 6.5 year period (43). They found no association between vitamin E and trace element plasma levels and the risk of hypertension. In women, a decreasing trend of hypertension risk was observed in the intervention group with vitamin C.
McInnes in his editorial to the above study (44) wrote:

"*The antioxidant enthusiasm of the 1990s, followed by the emergence of negative data from randomized controlled trials, reflects a healthy balance between basic clinical science and the development and evaluation of potentially preventive therapy... Further investigations are needed to understand the discrepancies between observational studies and randomized trials*."

LYCOPENE, BLOOD PRESSURE AND CARDIOVASCULAR DISEASES

Lycopene and some other tomato constituents are potent antioxidants. Their association with reducing atherosclerotic processes and cardiovascular (CV) morbidity has been described in the last decade. The oxidation-protecting effect of lycopene and tomatoes has been shown in both human and animal studies. A reduced oxidative modification of LDL may be one of the mechanisms by which lycopene reduces the risk of CAD and atherosclerotic progression (45).

Interest in lycopene has continued to grow in recent years, following the publication of epidemiologic and clinical studies concerning the association of high levels of lycopene and lower incidence of cardiovascular disease. Data from the Third National Health and Nutrition Examination Survey, 1988-1994 was analyzed for correlation between serum lycopene concentrations and sex, age, geographical location, race-ethnicity, education, alcohol, smoking, BMI, blood pressure, serum total cholesterol and triacylglycerol, and intakes of fat, tomatoes and tomato-based products in 3413 individuals aged 17-90 years. Sex, age, geographical region, socioeconomic status, serum total cholesterol, smoking, and intakes of fat, tomatoes, pizza, and pasta were significant determinants of serum lycopene concentrations in the United States (46).

Another study, using the same database, examined the association between microalbuminuria, a potent independent risk factor for CV disease, and circulating concentrations of vitamins A, C and E and carotenoids. Lycopene and total carotenoids were associated inversely with microalbuminuria (47). Similar results were documented in an Australian study (48).

Recently, Most MM. analyzed the phytochemical component of the DASH diet. Using the US Department of Agriculture food composition databases, the polyphenol, carotenoid, and phytosterol contents of the diets used in the DASH study were estimated. When compared with the control diet, the DASH diet is higher in flavonols, flavanones β-carotene, β-cryptoxanthin and lycopene. The author summarizes "It therefore is possible that the health benefits of the DASH diet are partially attributable to the phytochemicals and might extend beyond cardiovascular disease risk reduction." (49).

A multicenter case-control study was conducted to evaluate the relationship between antioxidant status assessed by biomarkers and acute myocardial infarction. The conclusion was that lycopene, or some substance highly correlated which is in a common food source, may contribute to the protective effect of vegetable consumption on myocardial infarction risk (50).

Another study investigated the relation between serum lycopene concentration and intima-media thickness of the common carotid artery of middle-aged men in Finland, the participants in the Kuopio Ischaemic Heart Disease Risk Factor study. A low serum lycopene concentration was found to be associated with a higher intima-media thickness. Increased thickness of the intima-media has been shown to predict coronary events; thus, lycopene intakes and serum concentrations may have clinical and public health relevance (51).

In spite of these promising results, prospective randomized studies evaluating the effect of different antioxidant vitamins on blood pressure levels are spare.

A small prospective interventional study compared the effects of short-term dietary supplementation with tomato juice, vitamin E, and vitamin C on susceptibility of LDL to oxidation and circulating levels of C-reactive protein (CRP) in patients with type 2 diabetes. In the intervention group an increased plasma lycopene was found together with higher CRP values, and a significantly higher resistance to oxidation of LDL. No change in BP was reported.

The Oxford Fruit and Vegetable Study Group evaluated the effects of fruit and vegetable consumption on plasma antioxidant concentrations and blood pressure. They found that plasma concentrations of different phyto-nutritients and vitamins (but not lycopene) increased significantly in the intervention group, compared to the regular diet group, while systolic and diastolic blood pressure decreased significantly. The authors concluded that effective intervention on fruit and vegetable consumption, plasma antioxidants, and blood pressure would be expected to reduce cardiovascular disease in the general population (14).

THE EXPERIENCE WITH LYCOPENE AND HYPERTENSION

Our long held interest in non-pharmacologic treatment of hypertension inspired us, a few years ago, to evaluate the BP lowering effect of several phyto-nutritients. After several short term pilot interventional studies, tomato extract seemed the most promising candidate. Tomato (Lycopersicon esculentum), is an important dietary source of antioxidants such as α-tocopherol and the carotenoids: β-carotene, phytoene, and phytofluene. Tomato is also the main dietary source of lycopene, the most potent antioxidant from the carotenoids (52).

Our primary hypothesis was that treatment with capsules containing tomato extract, rich in natural antioxidants, would produce a reduction in BP values in patients with grade-I untreated hypertension, without any associated disease. Through the choice of this mild hypertensive population, naïve to pharmacologic treatments, we hoped to include patients who could benefit from antioxidant treatment providing that they were still in the reversible phase of oxidative stress. A double-blind, placebo-controlled trial was designed as a pilot study to assess the changes in BP, oxidative stress and LDL oxidation in response to an 8-week treatment with tomato extract oleoresin capsules. * The results showed a drop of systolic blood pressure from 144 mmHg (SE±1.1) at the end of the placebo run-in period to 134 mmHg after 8 weeks of administration of tomato extract (SE±2, P<0.001), and diastolic blood pressure decreased from 87.4 mmHg (SE± 1.2) to 83.4 mmHg (SE ±1.2, P <0.05) respectively. After four weeks of the final placebo period systolic BP returned to the starting levels (144 mmHg ± 6.41) and diastolic BP increased significantly (85 ± 7.44 mmHg). On 24-hour ambulatory blood

*(Lyc-o-Mato□ made by LycoRed Natural Products Industries, Ltd).

pressure measurement (ABPM), average day-time SBP showed a significant reduction (from 137.44 ±11.78 mmHg) to normal range at the end of the intervention period (131.41 ± 14.04 mmHg, p=0.02). During the intervention period, lipid peroxidation products (AAPH-induced TBARS) declined from 4.58 ±1.34 to 3.81 ±1.58 nmol/mg (p=0.02) (53).

To further evaluate the effect of tomato extract on hypertension, we conducted another study involving grade I and II hypertension combined with pharmacological treatment. The aim of this study was to evaluate the effect of adding tomato extract to pharmacological treatment, in moderate hypertensives with uncontrolled BP levels, and to correlate this effect with plasma nitric oxide and serum lycopene levels. Fifty subjects with moderate hypertension, aged 46-66 years, treated with one or two antihypertensive medications, with BP equal or higher than 140/90 mmHg, without concomitant diseases, were recruited. After a routine base line evaluation, the study participants entered two double blind cross-over treatment periods of 6 weeks each with standardized tomato extract or identical placebo. The same tomato extract capsules were employed in the study, they provided a daily dose of 15 mg lycopene as well as β-carotene, vitamin E, phytoene, phytofluene and other phytonutrients.

Treatment with tomato extract reduced mean SBP from 144 mmHg at baseline to 131 mmHg, an average of 13 mmHg reduction and in DBP from 81 to 77 mmHg, an average of 4 mmHg reduction [Fig. 1].

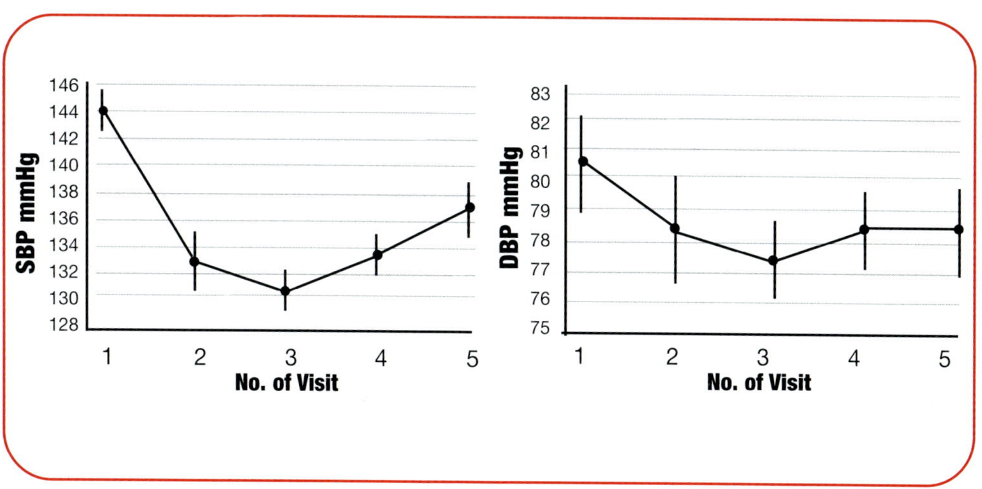

Fig 1: Systolic BP and diastolic BP changes on tomato extract treatment (visits 2-3) and on matching placebo (visits 4-5)

The mean plasma nitrate at baseline was 10.18 µM, tomato extract addition resulted an increase to 12.5 µM. During the placebo period plasma nitrate levels remained close to baseline 9.7 µM. The changes in plasma lycopene, were in correlation with the drop of BP during the treatment period with tomato extract and with plasma nitrate levels [Fig. 2] (54).

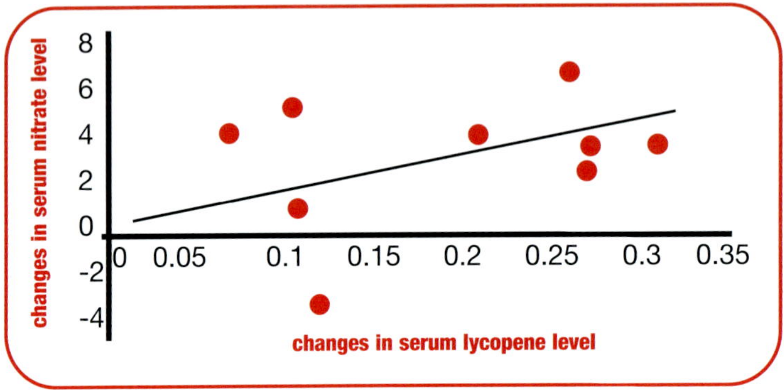

Fig 2: Correlation between changes of serum nitrate and serum lycopene, during treatment with tomato extract (9 patients)

CONCLUSION

The positive results of these trials are encouraging; however, these are relatively small studies, with patient population comprised low-risk grade-1 hypertension only. The course of therapy was relatively short, and it is not clear whether the beneficial effect of tomato extract will persist with prolonged administration. It is reasonable to assume that these low-risk patients who have only minor or no vascular damage will be more responsive to the intervention than patients with higher-grade hypertension and more advanced vascular disease and multiple drug therapy. However, according to our knowledge this is the first properly designed and conducted clinical trial to evaluate the effect of tomato extract, lycopene on BP of hypertensive patients. A drop in BP from grade-1 hypertension range to high normal range, such as achieved in our study, is clinically significant. Maintaining patients in a normotensive state and preventing progression to a higher-grade of hypertension may postpone or even avert the need for antihypertensive drug therapy. The results of the second study suggest that the addition of antioxidant-rich tomato extract to the pharmacological treatment of moderate hypertensives may be used as an adjuvant to anti-hypertensive therapy. In this trial tomato extract was shown not only to reduce BP but to increase plasma nitrate level, a measure of improved endothelial function. Whether a longer treatment could produce a beneficial effect on cardiovascular risk factors and prevention of target organ damage should be evaluated in the future.

REFERENCES:

1. Hajjar, I. and T. A. Kotchen (2003). "Trends in prevalence, awareness, treatment, and control of hypertension in the United States, 1988-2000." Jama 290(2): 199-206.
2. Fields, L. E., V. L. Burt, et al. (2004). "The burden of adult hypertension in the United States 1999 to 2000: a rising tide." Hypertension 44(4): 398-404.
3. Thrift, A. G., J. J. McNeil, et al. (1996). "Risk factors for cerebral hemorrhage in the era of well-controlled hypertension. Melbourne Risk Factor Study (MERFS) Group." Stroke 27(11):2020-5.
4. Greenland, P., M. D. Knoll, et al. (2003). "Major risk factors as antecedents of fatal and nonfatal coronary heart disease events." Jama 290(7): 891-7.
5. Chobanian, A. V., G. L. Bakris, et al. (2003). "The Seventh Report of the Joint National Committee on Prevention, Detection, Evaluation, and Treatment of High Blood Pressure: the JNC 7 report." Jama 289(19): 2560-72.
6. (2003). "2003 European Society of Hypertension-European Society of Cardiology guidelines for the management of arterial hypertension." J Hypertens 21(6): 1011-53.
7. Lewington, S., R. Clarke, et al. (2002). "Age-specific relevance of usual blood pressure to vascular mortality: a meta-analysis of individual data for one million adults in 61 prospective studies." Lancet 360(9349): 1903-13.
8. Pastor-Barriuso, R., J. R. Banegas, et al. (2003). "Systolic blood pressure, diastolic blood pressure, and pulse pressure: an evaluation of their joint effect on mortality." Ann Intern Med 139(9): 731-9.
9. Jackson, R., C. M. Lawes, et al. (2005). "Treatment with drugs to lower blood pressure and blood cholesterol based on an individual's absolute cardiovascular risk." Lancet 365(9457): 434-41.
10. Appel, L. J., M. W. Brands, et al. (2006). "Dietary approaches to prevent and treat hypertension: a scientific statement from the American Heart Association." Hypertension 47(2): 296-308.
11. Moore, T. J., P. R. Conlin, et al. (2001). "DASH (Dietary Approaches to Stop Hypertension) diet is effective treatment for stage 1 isolated systolic hypertension." Hypertension 38(2): 155-8.
12. Hennekens, C. H., J. E. Buring, et al. (1996). "Lack of effect of long-term supplementation with beta carotene on the incidence of malignant neoplasms and cardiovascular disease." N Engl J Med 334(18): 1145-9.
13. Yusuf, S., G. Dagenais, et al. (2000). "Vitamin E supplementation and cardiovascular events in high-risk patients. The Heart Outcomes Prevention Evaluation Study Investigators." N Engl J Med 342(3): 154-60
14. John, J. H., S. Ziebland, et al. (2002). "Effects of fruit and vegetable consumption on plasma antioxidant concentrations and blood pressure: a randomized controlled trial." Lancet 359(9322): 1969-74.
15. Madamanchi, N. R., A. Vendrov, et al. (2005). "Oxidative stress and vascular disease." Arterioscler Thromb Vasc Biol 25(1): 29-38.
16. Cai, H. and D. G. Harrison (2000). "Endothelial dysfunction in cardiovascular diseases: the role of oxidant stress." Circ Res 87(10): 840-4.
17. Endemann, D. H. and E. L. Schiffrin (2004). "Endothelial dysfunction." J Am Soc Nephrol 15(8): 1983-92.

18. Griendling, K. K. and D. G. Harrison (1999). "Dual role of reactive oxygen species in vascular growth." Circ Res 85(6): 562-3.
19. Shokoji, T., A. Nishiyama, et al. (2003). "Renal sympathetic nerve responses to tempol in spontaneously hypertensive rats." Hypertension 41(2): 266-73.
20. Virdis, A., M. F. Neves, et al. (2004). "Role of NAD(P)H oxidase on vascular alterations in angiotensin II-infused mice." J Hypertens 22(3): 535-42.
21. Wilcox, C. S. (2005). "Oxidative stress and nitric oxide deficiency in the kidney: a critical link to hypertension?" Am J Physiol Regul Integr Comp Physiol 289(4): R913-35.
22. Lip, G. Y., E. Edmunds, et al. (2002). "Oxidative stress in malignant and non-malignant phase hypertension." J Hum Hypertens 16(5): 333-6.
23. Kumar, K. V. and U. N. Das (1993). "Are free radicals involved in the pathobiology of human essential hypertension?" Free Radic Res Commun 19(1): 59-66.
24. Redon, J., M. R. Oliva, et al. (2003). "Antioxidant activities and oxidative stress byproducts in human hypertension." Hypertension 41(5): 1096-101.
25. Antioxidants Block Angiotensin II-Induced Increases in Blood Pressure and Endothelin Maria Clara Ortiz; Melissa C. Manriquez; Juan C. Romero; Luis A. Juncos Hypertension. 2001 Sep;38(3 Pt 2):655-9
26. Katusic, Z. S. (1996). "Superoxide anion and endothelial regulation of arterial tone." Free Radic Biol Med 20(3): 443-8.
27. Rajagopalan, S., S. Kurz, et al. (1996). "Angiotensin II-mediated hypertension in the rat increases vascular superoxide production via membrane NADH/NADPH oxidase activation. Contribution to alterations of vasomotor tone." J Clin Invest 97(8): 1916-23.
28. Hazan-Halevy, I., T. Levy, et al. (2005). "Stimulation of NADPH oxidase by angiotensin II in human neutrophils is mediated by ERK, p38 MAP-kinase and cytosolic phospholipase A2." J Hypertens 23(6): 1183-90.
29. Lockette, W., Y. Otsuka, et al. (1986). "The loss of endothelium-dependent vascular relaxation in hypertension." Hypertension 8(6 Pt 2): II61-6.
30. Solzbach, U., B. Hornig, et al. (1997). "Vitamin C improves endothelial dysfunction of epicardial coronary arteries in hypertensive patients." Circulation 96(5): 1513-9.
31. Heistad, D. D. (2006). "Oxidative Stress and Vascular Disease. 2005 Duff Lecture." Arterioscler Thromb Vasc Biol.
32. Schiffrin, E. L., J. B. Park, et al. (2002). "Effect of crossing over hypertensive patients from a beta-blocker to an angiotensin receptor antagonist on resistance artery structure and on endothelial function." J Hypertens 20(1): 71-8.
33. Conlin, P. R., D. Chow, et al. (2000). "The effect of dietary patterns on blood pressure control in hypertensive patients: results from the Dietary Approaches to Stop Hypertension (DASH) trial." Am J Hypertens 13(9): 949-55.
34. Curin, Y., R. Andriantsitohaina, et al. (2005). "Polyphenols as potential therapeutical agents against cardiovascular diseases Oxidative Stress and Vascular Disease. 2005 Duff Lecture Renal Mitochondrial Dysfunction In Spontaneously Hypertensive Rats Is Attenuated By Losartan But Not By Amlodipine." Pharmacol Rep. 57(Suppl): 97-107.
35. Moran, J. P., L. Cohen, et al. (1993). "Plasma ascorbic acid concentrations relate inversely to blood pressure in human subjects." Am J Clin Nutr 57(2): 213-7.
36. Bates, C. J., C. M. Walmsley, et al. (1998). "Does vitamin C reduce blood pressure? Results of a large study of people aged 65 or older." J Hypertens 16(7): 925-32.
37. Chen, J., J. He, et al. (2002). "Serum antioxidant vitamins and blood pressure in the

United States population." Hypertension 40(6): 810-6.
38. Fotherby, M. D., J. C. Williams, et al. (2000). "Effect of vitamin C on ambulatory blood pressure and plasma lipids in older persons." J Hypertens 18(4): 411-5.
39. Ness, A. and J. Sterne (2000). "Hypertension and ascorbic acid." Lancet 355(9211): 1271; author reply 1273-4.
40. Rolla, G., L. Brussino, et al. (2000). "Hypertension and ascorbic acid." Lancet 355(9211): 1271-2; author reply 1273-4.
41. Kim, M. K., S. Sasaki, et al. (2002). "Lack of long-term effect of vitamin C supplementation on blood pressure." Hypertension 40(6): 797-803.
42. (2002). "MRC/BHF Heart Protection Study of antioxidant vitamin supplementation in 20,536 high-risk individuals: a randomised placebo-controlled trial." Lancet 360(9326): 23-33.
43. Czernichow, S., S. Bertrais, et al. (2005). "Effect of supplementation with antioxidants upon long-term risk of hypertension in the SU.VI.MAX study: association with plasma antioxidant levels." J Hypertens 23(11): 2013-8.
44. McInnes, G. T. (2005). "Antioxidants and hypertension: another false dawn?" J Hypertens 23(11): 1963-6.
45. Agarwal, S. and A. V. Rao (1998). "Tomato lycopene and low density lipoprotein oxidation: a human dietary intervention study." Lipids 33(10): 981-4
46. Ganji, V. and M. R. Kafai (2005). "Population determinants of serum lycopene concentrations in the United States: data from the Third National Health and Nutrition Examination Survey, 1988-1994." J Nutr 135(3): 567-72.
47. Ford, E. S., W. H. Giles, et al. (2005). "Microalbuminuria and concentrations of antioxidants among US adults." Am J Kidney Dis 45(2): 248-55.
48. Rowley, K., K. O'Dea, et al. (2003). "Low plasma concentrations of diet-derived antioxidants in association with microalbuminuria in Indigenous Australian populations." Clin Sci (Lond) 105(5): 569-75.
49. Most, M. M. (2004). "Estimated phytochemical content of the dietary approaches to stop hypertension (DASH) diet is higher than in the Control Study Diet." J Am Diet Assoc 104(11): 1725-7.
50. Kohlmeier, L., J. D. Kark, et al. (1997). "Lycopene and myocardial infarction risk in the EURAMIC Study." Am J Epidemiol 146(8): 618-26.
51. Rissanen, T. H., S. Voutilainen, et al. (2003). "Serum lycopene concentrations and carotid atherosclerosis: the Kuopio Ischaemic Heart Disease Risk Factor Study." Am J Clin Nutr 77(1): 133-8.
52. Gerster, H. (1997). "The potential role of lycopene for human health." J Am Coll Nutr 16(2): 109-26.
53. Engelhard, Y. N., B. Gazer, et al. (2006). "Natural antioxidants from tomato extract reduce blood pressure in patients with grade-1 hypertension: a double-blind, placebo-controlled pilot study." Am Heart J 151(1): 100.
54. Paran, E., Y. N. Engelhard, et al.(2005). "Effect of standardized tomato extract on blood pressure, endothelial function and plasma lycopen levels in treated hypertensive patients" Am J Hypertens 18(5): 213A

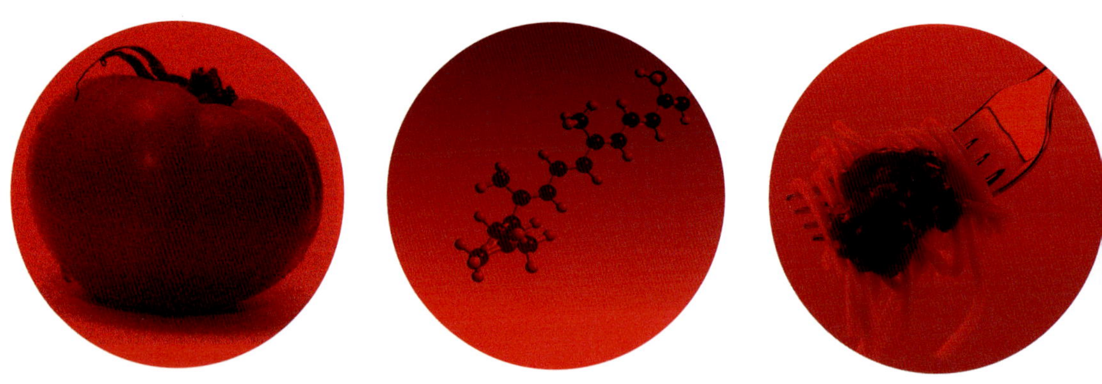

Reversing Male Infertility with Tomato Lycopene

Dr. N.K. Mohanty
Dept. of Urology
V.M. Medical College & Safdarjang Hospital
New Delhi
India

Abstract

Infertility has had a major impact on our society since the dawn of humanity. Unlike other civilizations, infertility in the early Egyptian society was not viewed as a divine punishment but was considered an illness which merited proper diagnosis and treatment. Nowadays, despite enormous progress in research most of the blame for infertility until recently was placed on the females. In the last one and a half decades, scientific advances and a better understanding of sperm physiology, anatomy and functions have increased our knowledge relating to male infertility. Close to 15% of couples are reported to suffer from infertility and 5-10% of all males are infertile or sub-fertile. A recent WHO study showed that male infertility accounts for half of all involuntarily childless couples. (Fig.1)

Female
39%
Male
20%
No Cause
15%
Male & Female
26%

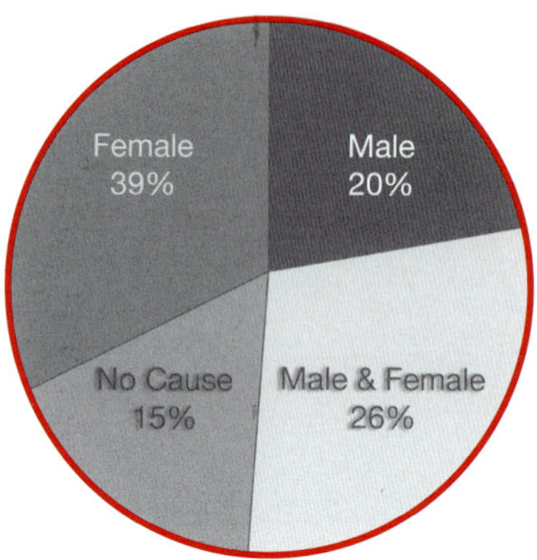

Figure 1: Causes of infertility among males and females

Although many environmental, physiological and genetic factors contribute to male infertility (Table 1), defective sperm function is thought to be the most common cause.

Factors in Male Infertility	%
Idiopathic Infertility	31.6%
Varicocele	25.0%
Hypogonadism	10.5%
Infection	9.9%
Maldescended Testis	7.8%
Immunological factors	3.0%
Endocrine	2.0%
Systemic/General disease	4.5%
Obstruction to Vas	4.0%
Gynaecomastia	1.1%
Testicular tumors	0.6%

Table 1: Factors contributing to male infertility

In addition to the above factors, lifestyle, diet, heat, alcohol and smoking can also contribute to male infertility. Free radical induced oxidative damage to spermatozoa is one such condition which has recently been gaining considerable attention for its role in inducing defective sperm function and male infertility.

BIOLOGY OF REACTIVE OXYGEN SPECIES (ROS)

ROS are ubiquitous in aerobic biologic systems. They effect diverse cellular functions and cellular differentiation as well as cellular aging (enzyme inactivation, DNA break, lipid oxidation, tumerogenesis). Pathological disorders associated with ROS stem from imbalances between their production and scavenging (Figure 2).

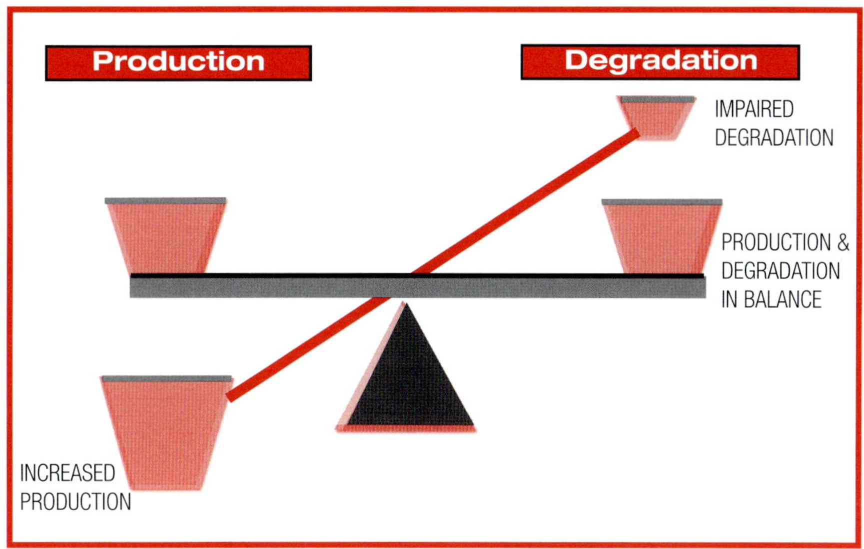

Figure 2: Production and Degradation of ROS Associated with Pathological Disorders. A balance between production and degradation of ROS siginifies normal pathology.

The reactivity of various species of ROS and their sources in semen are shown in Tables 2 and 3.

	Strength	Potential targets
O_2	+	SHgpe, NADH
H_2O_2	++	DNA, SHgpe
-OH	++++	Lipids, DNA, SHgpe
$-NO^-$	++	Metals, SHgpe, ROS

Table 2: Reactivity and Potential Targets of ROS

1. Leukocytes (WBC)
2. Spermatozoa

- WBC concentration correlates with ROS levels in whole semen. (Fig.3)
- The generation of ROS by human spermatozoa occurs spontaneously under aerobic conditions. Defective sperm function (e.g. motility) is associated with the accumulation of lipid peroxides.
- Retained cytoplasm (RC) mid-piece area correlates with ROS production and this can alter sperm dysfunction (motility, fertilization *in vitro*).

Table 3: Sources of ROS in Semen

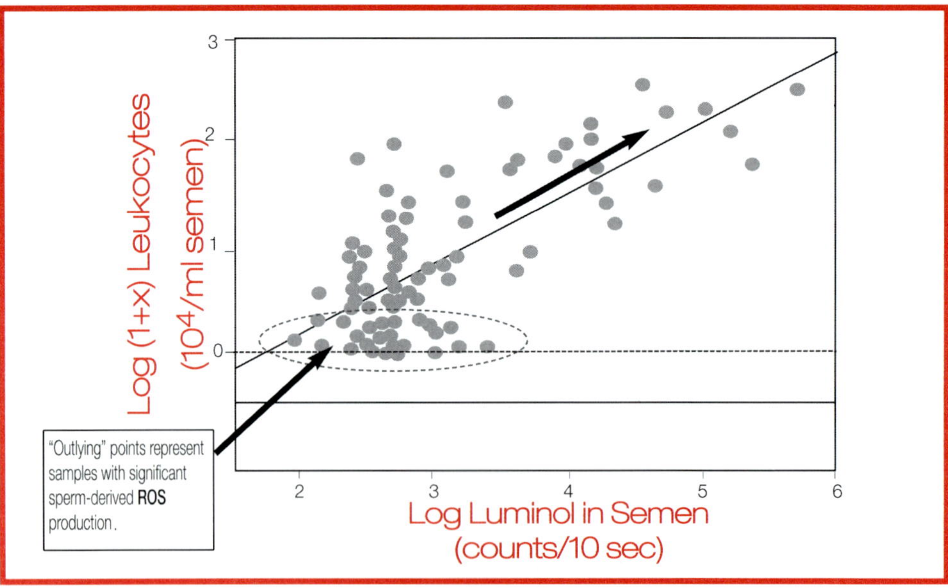

Figure 3: Relationship between leukocyte concentration and ROS levels in whole semen

REACTIVE OXYGEN SPECIES (ROS) ON SPERM FUNCTION

The concept that free radicals can influence male infertility has received substantial scientific support (2). The proposed mechanism for loss of sperm function upon oxidative stress has been shown to involve excessive generation of reactive oxygen species (ROS) (3). Presence of leukocytes in semen has been associated with severe male factor infertility (4,5). There has been much speculation as to whether the origin of ROS in semen is from spermatozoa or from infiltrating leukocytes (6,7). Greater sperm motility was observed in semen samples with lesser amounts of detectable ROS than in those with higher levels of ROS (8).

All living aerobic cells are normally exposed to ROS but cellular damage takes place as a result of improper balance between ROS generation and existing scavenging activities. The scavenging potential in gonads and seminal fluid is normally maintained by adequate levels of antioxidants, like superoxide dismutase (SOD), catalase and glutathionate (GSH). A situation in which there is a shift in the ROS balance because of either excess ROS or diminished antioxidants, can result oxidative stress status (OSS). OSS has been shown to be a major cause of male infertility. (Fig. 4)

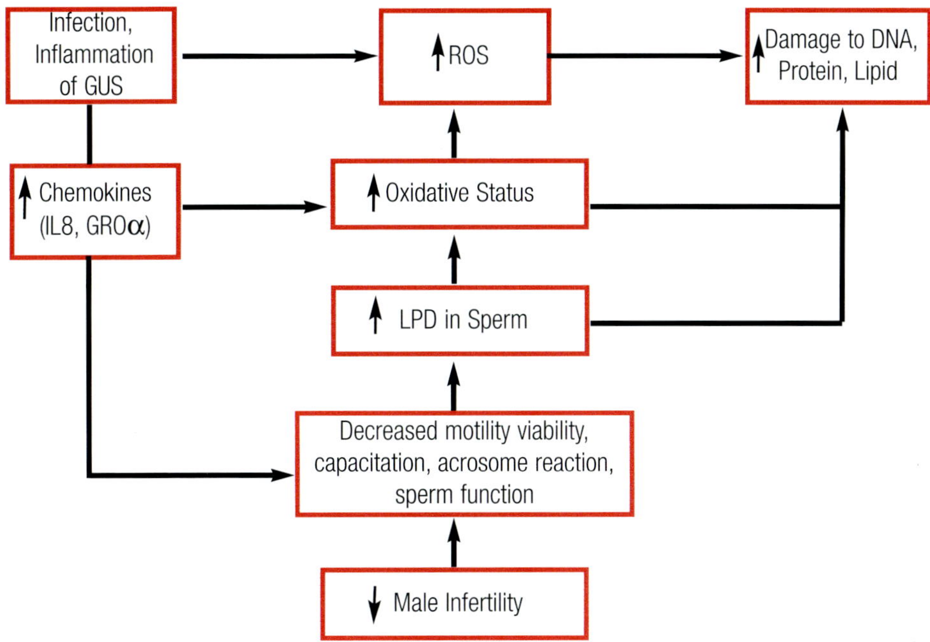

Figure 4: Relationship Between Oxidative Stress Status and Male Infertility

ROS AND NORMAL SPERM FUNCTION

The human spermatozoa cell wall is rich in polyunsaturated fatty acid which is susceptible to ROS. Lipid peroxidation of sperm membrane due to OSS results in sperm damage and sperm apoptosis leading to infertility (9). Several forms of sperm DNA damage are caused by ROS e.g. chromatin cross linking, hromosome deletion, DNA strand breaks & base oxidation, ATP depletion, and oxidation of proteins/ SH group (10).

FACTORS AFFECTING ROS LEVELS AND ACTIVITY

Several factors influence the antioxidant status and the levels of ROS in the seminal fluid. The significance of these factors are shown in Table 4.

Factor	Significance
Idiopathic infertility	In men with idiopathic infertility there is significantly higher seminal fluid ROS level & lower antioxidant properties than in the controls (11).
Genital tract infection	Leukocytospermia results in increased ROS level & cytokines resulting in sperm DNA damage. The study shows that the level of oxidative DNA damage marker, 8-hydroxyl-2-deoxyguanosine (8-OHdG) was significantly elevated in infertile males with infection (12).
Varicocele	Elevated levels of ROS has been detected in infertile patients with varicocele with reduced levels of both seminal & blood plasma antioxidants (13). Higher sperm DNA fragmentation index (DFI) has been detected in infertile men with varicocele than their healthy counterparts (14). Another cause of sperm DNA damage in patients with varicocele is apoptosis. Levels of apoptosis are higher in ejaculated spermatozoa from infertile males with varicocele than in spermatozoa from healthy males.
Teratozoospermia	ROS production is highest in immature spermatozoa. Teratozoospermics have an abundance of such immature spermatozoa carrying surplus residual cytoplasm which generates endogenous ROS mediated by cytosolic enzyme glucose-6-phosphate dehydrogenase (15).
Asthenospermia	Increased ROS damages sperm DNA which affects sperm motility by damaging the axonemal structure (16).
Azoospermia	Increased ROS not only damages sperm but also results in apoptosis. This may interrupt the spermatogenic cascade, resulting in azoospermia.
Aging	Some forms of infertility are caused by age-related degenerative disorders of the testis. Presence of immature spermatozoa with retained cytoplasm in aging males may release increased ROS. Decreased vascularity, increased spermatogenic failure & reduced sperm output occur in aging males.

Table 4: Factors Effecting Levels and Activity of ROS

MANAGEMENT OF MALE INFERTILITY

Because OSS is the result of imbalance between ROS levels and total antioxidant capacity (TAC) of seminal plasma, it is important to assess both these factors while evaluating OSS of a given semen sample. The chemiluminescence assay is one of the most common methods used to detect free radicals. Samples should be analyzed within one hour of sample collection. Values of more than 1 x 10^6/ml photons per minute are considered high.

In clinical practice the DNA fragmentation index (DFI) not only distinguishes fertile men from those who are infertile but also identifies samples that are compatible with *in vivo* and *in vitro* pregnancy.

Recent research and studies have shown that:

- 40-80% of idiopathic infertile males have high levels of free oxygen radicals.
- Semen ROS levels correlate negatively with sperm motility (17). (Fig. 5)

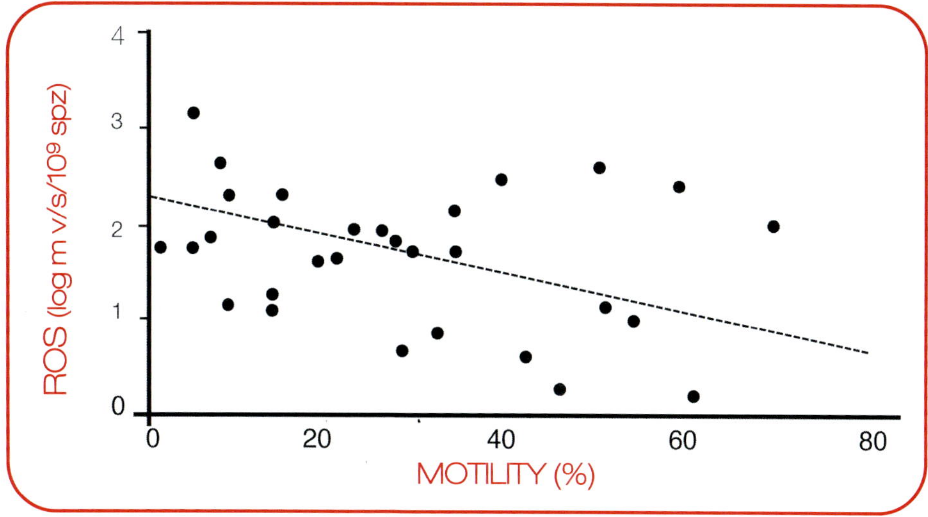

Fig. 5: Association between semen ROS levels and sperm motility

- Men with high levels of free oxygen radicals have sevenfold less chance of initiating pregnancy.
- Infertile males have decreased antioxidant defence in seminal plasma.
- High level of semen ROS are associated with low pregnancy rates *in vivo* (18). (Fig. 6)

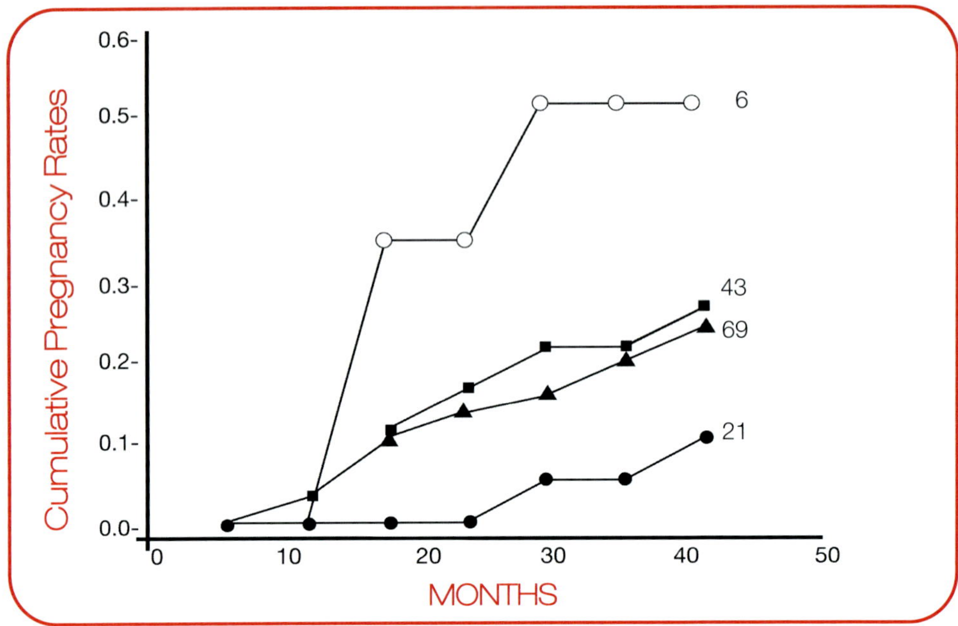

Fig. 6: Association between semen ROS levels and sperm motility

- Idiopathic infertile males have low levels of antioxidants.
- Lycopene is found in high concentration in both the testis and prostate (19).
- Testis lycopene levels – 20nmol per gram of tissue.
- Serum lycopene levels – 0.5nmol per ml.
- Addition of antioxidants brought beneficial effect in preventing loss of sperm motility & inhibiting lipid peroxidation (20).
- Antioxidants can improve sperm function and correct male infertility (20).
- One of the most common abnormalities associated with male infertility is the presence of free radical in the ejaculate.
- Decreased antioxidant capacity is associated with impaired sperm function.
- The levels of lycopene was significantly decreased in seminal plasma of infertile men as compared to fertile men.
- Subsequent to SOD, only levels of lycopene were found to be depleted in the seminal plasma of infertile men.

TREATMENT OF MALE INFERTILITY

WHO Guidelines for Normal Semen Analysis Parameters are shown in Table 5.

WHO Guidelines for Normal Semen Parameters	
Volume	1.5-5.0ml
pH	Alkaline
Sperm concentration	> 20million/ml
Functional sperm conc.	> 3 million/ml
Sperm motility	> 50%
Sperm motility index	> 80%
Sperm morphology	> 30% normal forms
Leukocyte density	< 1million/ml
Fructose	+ve

Table 5: WHO Guidelines for Normal Semen Parameters

Male infertile patients with defective spermatozoa due to OSS from increased ROS have to be treated with oral antioxidants in order to reduce the ROS level because low levels of oxidative stress *in vitro* enhances sperm hyperactivation, sperm capacitation, acrosome reaction, sperm-egg binding, sperm-egg fusion and fertilization.

Antioxidants that act to protect sperm from ROS are shown in Table 6.

Antioxidants that Protect Sperm from ROS Damage
SOD
Catalase
Glutathione peroxidase
Taurine/ Hypotaurine
Vitamin-C & E
Urate
Lycopene

Table 6: Antioxidants that protect sperm from ROS damage.

ROLE OF ANTIOXIDANTS IN SEMEN

The role of antioxidants in semen is to:

- Protect normal sperm from ROS producing sperm.
- Protect normal sperm from WBC-derived ROS.
- Suppress premature sperm maturation,

The sites of action of these antioxidants include:

- Male reproduction tract.
- Female reproductive tract.

The treatment of oxidative stress-mediated male infertility therefore includes both disease-specific and antioxidant therapy.

SOME ASPECTS OF DISEASE-SPECIFIC THERAPY

1. Appropriate antibiotic therapy for genital tract infection.
2. Surgical management for varicocele to improve sperm morphology and decrease the percentage of spermatozoa with retained cytoplasm.
3. Lifestyle changes to reduce oxidative stress such as avoiding alcohol, tobacco smoking and performing regular physical exercise to reduce stress.

Whereas the antioxidant therapy includes in vitro therapy which is effective in preserving serum motility and oral supplementation with primary antioxidants such as lycopene.

LYCOPENE

Lycopene is a component of the human redox defence mechanism against free radicals. It is a primary antioxidant, one of the 650 carotenoids, found abundantly in tomatoes, guavas & pink watermelons.

Lycopene constitutes approximately 50% of all carotenoids found in human blood serum. As a person grows older, the lycopene serum values decrease.

Lycopene has been shown in experiments to have the highest oxygen-quenching capacity (strongest antioxidant). It is twice as powerful as β-carotene at neutralizing free radicals and 100 times more potent than vitamin E. This antioxidant property protects the cells from DNA damage. The mean plasma level of lycopene ranges from 0.22 to 1.06nmol/ml.

The evidence for the role of lycopene in male infertility has been the subject of several recent studies. The highlights from these studies include the following:

-The human organism cannot synthesize lycopene and therefore obtains it from the food we eat.

- Level of lycopene in seminal plasma was low in immuno infertile men as compared to fertile men .

- Levels of ROS can be reduced by augmenting this scavenging capacity of the seminal plasma with antioxidants.

- Significantly lower levels of lycopene in the seminal plasma of immuno infertile men as compared to fertile men (19ng/ml vs 42ng/ml).

- Oral lycopene (2mg twice daily) showed maximum improvement in sperm concentration in the management of idiopathic male infertility.

- *In vitro* and *in vivo* lycopene supplementation protects cells from induced oxidative damage. Lipid peroxidation is reduced by 80%, DNA oxidation is reduced by 75% (Fig.7).

- Oral lycopene supplementation protects against *ex vivo* induced lymphocyte DNA oxidation. DNA fragmentation is reduced by 40%. (Fig. 7).

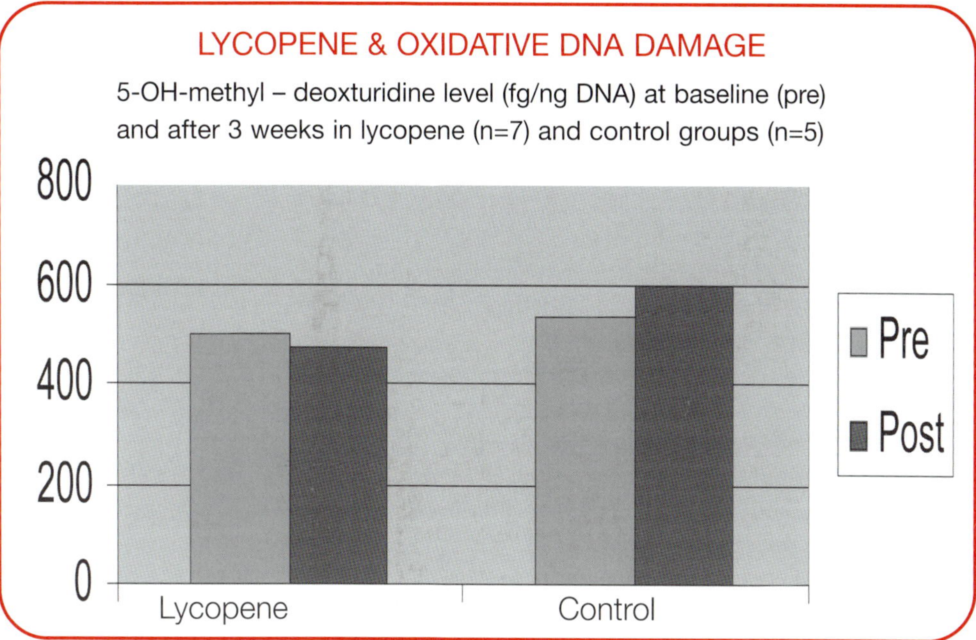

Fig. 7: Effect of lycopene supplementation on oxidative DNA damage in human subjects

- Lycopene in raw tomato is less available than that obtained from processed tomato products and its bioavailability increases when it is consumed with small amount of lipids.

- The recommended daily allowance for lycopene is 5-10mg/day.

- Lycopene in its biological environment in combination with low doses of Vitamin A, E, C, Zinc and Selenium as bioactive phytonutrients provides full antioxidant effect in scavenging ROS and preventing damage to sperm.

- Idiopathic infertile males treated with lycopene demonstrated improved semen characteristics, fertilization in vitro and it thus contributed to a higher pregnancy rate.

CONCLUSION AND FUTURE STUDIES

Spermatozoa possess an inherent but limited capacity to generate ROS which help in the fertilization process. Controlled generation of ROS has a physiologically beneficial role in spermatozoal functions such as hyper activation and capacitation acrosome reactions, but increased levels of ROS lead to oxidative stress status (OSS) which will result in defective sperm function, sperm apoptosis and male infertility. Therefore a balance between benefits and risk for ROS and antioxidants is mandatory for the survival and normal functioning of spermatozoa.

The role of lycopene in the management of male infertility is very promising. More research work should be undertaken with randomized trials to:

- Evaluate lycopene levels and markers of oxidative stress in sperm and semen of infertile and fertile males.

- Correlate sperm and semen lycopene levels with dietary intake of lycopene in infertile males.

- Study the effect of lycopene supplementation on semen lycopene level and sperm parameters in infertile males.

Lycopene supplementation via increased natural dietary intake of foods rich in lycopene such as processed tomato products or natural lycopene extracts, for infertile males having no other definite treatable cause for their infertility is not only safe but also greatly improves their sperm count, motility and improves their sperm morphology to optimum levels thereby significantly increasing their chances to become proud fathers.

REFERENCES:

1. M. Hull, C.Glazener, N.Kelly, D.Conway, P.Foster, R.Hunton, C.Coulson, P.Lambert, E.Watt & K.Desai : Population study of causes, treatment and outcome of infertility. Br Med J 291, 1693-7 (1985).
2. C.Gagnon, A.Iwasaki, E de Lamirande, N.Kovalski : Reactive oxygen species and human spermatozoa. Ann N Y Acad Sci 637, 436-44 (1991).
3. R.J.Aitken, J.S.Clarkson : Cellular basis of defective sperm function and its association with the genesis of reactive oxygen species by human spermatozoa. J Reprod Fertil 81, 459-69 (1987).
4. R.J.Aitken, D.Buckingham, K.West, F.C.Wu, K.Zikopoulos & D.W. Richardson : Differential contribution of leukocytes and spermatozoa to the generation of reactive oxygen species in the ejaculates of oligozoospermic patients and fertile donors. J Reprod Fertil 94, 451-62 (1992).
5. H.Wolff & D.J.Anderson : Immunohistologic characterization and quantitation of leucocyte subpopulations in human semen. Fertil Steril 49, 497-504 (1988).
6. E.Kessopoulou, M.J.Tomlinson, C.L.Barratt, A.E.Boltron & I.D.Cooke : Origin of reactive oxygen species in human semen : spermatozoa or leucocytes? J Reprod Fertil 94, 463-70 (1992).
7. C.Krausz, C.Mills, S.Rogers, S.L.Tan, R.J.Aitken : Stimulation of oxidant generation by human sperm suspensions using phorbol esters and formyl peptides : relationships with motility and fertilization in vitro. Fertil Steril 62, 599-605 (1994).
8. A.Iwasaki & C.Gagnon : Formation of reactive oxygen species in spermatozoa of infertile patients. Fertil Steril 57, 409-416 (1992).
9. J.G.Alvarez, J.C.Touchstone, L.Blasco & B.T.Stoery : Spontaneous lipid peroxidation and production of hydrogen peroxide and superoxide in human spermatozoa. Superoxide dismutase as major enzyme protectant against against oxygen toxicity. J Androl 8, 338-348 (1987).
10. Ashok Agarwal & Tamer M.Said : Oxidative stress, DNA damage and apoptosis in male infertility : a clinical approach. BJU Int 2005 Mar; Vol.95(4): 503-7.

11. Pasqualotto F, Sharma R, Kobayashi H, Nelson D, Thomas A Jr, Agarwal A. Oxidative stress in normospermic men undergoing infertility evaluation. J Androl 2001; 73:459-64.
12. Kodama H, Yamaguchi R, Fukuda J, Kasai H, Tanaka T. Increased oxidative deoxyribonucleic acid damage in the spermatozoa of infertile male patients. Fertil Steril 1997; 68: 519-24.
13. Barbieri E, Hidalgo M, Venegas A, Smith R, Lissi E. Varicocele-associated decrease in antioxidant defenses. J Androl 1999; 20:713-7.
14. Saleh R, Agarwal A, Sharma R, Said T, Sikka S, Thomas A Jr. Evaluation of nuclear DNA damage in spermatozoa from infertile men with varicocele. Fertil Steril 2003; 80:1431-6.
15. Aitken R. The Amoroso lecture. The human spermatozoon — a cell in crisis? J Reprod Fertil 1999; 115 : 1-7.
16. Saleh A, Agarwal A. Oxidative stress and male infertility : from research bench to clinical practice. J Androl 2002; 23: 737-52.
17. Agarwal A, Nallella K, Allamaneni S, Said T. Role of antioxidants in treatment of male infertility : an overview of the literature. Reprod Biomedicine Online 2004; 8:616-27.
18. Irvine DS et al. DNA integrity in human spermatozoa : relationships with semen quality. J Androl 2000; 21:33-34.
19. Lewis EM et al. Comparison of individual antioxidants of sperm and seminal plasma in fertile and infertile men. Fertil Steril 1997; 67: 142-147.
20. Shen H et al. Detection of oxidative DNA damage in human sperm and its association with sperm function and male infertility. Free Radic Biol Med 2000; 28:529-536.

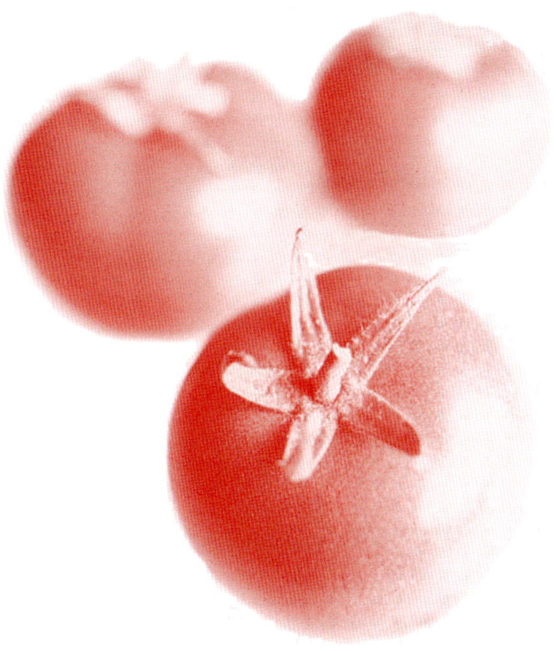

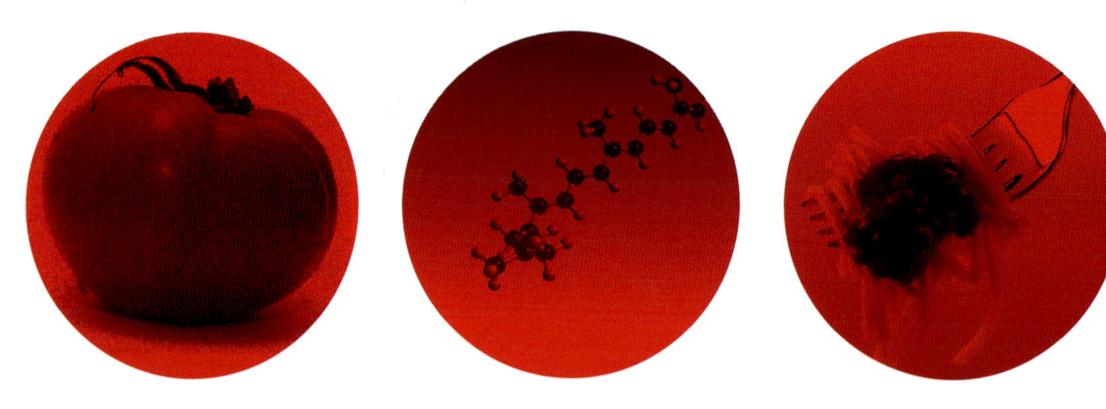

Tomato Lycopene in Photoprotection and Skin Care

Prof. Dr. W. Stahl
Institute of Biochemistry and Molecular Biology I
Heinrich-Heine-University
Duesseldorf, Germany

Abstract

UV-irradiation of human skin leads to photooxidative damage associated with adverse effects on skin health and appearance. Endogenous supply of the skin with micronutrients may contribute to photoprotection. Carotenoids are important components of the light-protecting system in plants and prevent UV damage in humans. The protective properties have been attributed to the pronounced antioxidant effects of these compounds. Lycopene is the major carotenoid of the tomato and a very efficient antioxidant. Human intervention studies provide evidence that skin can be protected against UV-dependent lesions by supplying lycopene or a lycopene-rich diet.

1. INTRODUCTION

Our skin is the largest organ of the body and an important barrier protecting against pathogenic organisms and toxic agents. It mediates exchanges with the surroundings (like temperature regulation and sensation) but also plays a major role in insulation. Skin represents a storage center for lipids and water and is the location of UV-dependent vitamin D synthesis. Histologically, skin (*cutis*) is divided into two main layers, epidermis and dermis (*corium*), attached to underlying subcutaneous connective and adipose tissue. The principal cells of the epidermis are the keratinocytes, which are continuously generated at the basement membrane and migrate to the skin surface. Other epidermal cells are the melanocytes synthesizing the pigment melanin and Langerhans cells participating in the cutaneous immune response. Dead and peeling cells, mainly keratinocytes, filled with mature keratin form the outer horny skin layer *(stratum corneum*).

Dermis consists of dense fibrous connective tissue, with collagen the predominant component, containing blood vessels for nutrient supply. Nerve fibers, lymphatic vessels, sebaceous glands and sweat gland channels are embedded in the epidermis. Mainly, the dermis is responsible for the skin's structural integrity, elasticity and resilience. Age-related structural changes, like the formation of wrinkles, arise and develop in the dermis.

The subcutaneous layer contains sweat glands, some hair follicles, blood vessels, and fat. Adipocytes are the predominant type of cells in the subcutaneous tissue.
Light penetrates the skin and interacts with biological structures at the different layers. The penetration depth of light depends on structural features and pigmentation, which influence absorption, reflection, and scattering; the longer the wavelength, the deeper the light penetration (1, 2). UVA and visible light reach the dermis and to some extent also the subcutis, whereas UVB practically does not pass beyond the epidermal layer. UVB combines tissue targeting and damaging properties in such a way that most of the severe consequences of UV exposure are attributed to this wavelength range. However, UVA radiation is involved in processes of photoaging and photocarcinogenesis, playing a major role in the pathogenesis of photodermatoses (3). There is also evidence from *in vitro* and *in vivo* studies that infrared radiation may play a role in photoaging (4). Upon light exposure, a cascade of photo-induced chemical and biological reactions takes place in the target tissue (5-9). Reactive oxygen species (ROS) are generated in photooxidative processes and damage molecules and cellular structures. The chemical reaction cascade leads to cellular biochemical responses including modified gene expression, impact on kinase-dependent regulatory pathways, immune and inflammatory events, or induction of apoptosis. Photooxidative damage affects cellular lipids, proteins and DNA and is involved in the pathobiochemistry of erythema formation, premature aging of the skin, development of photodermatoses, and skin cancer (10).

2. NUTRITION AND SKIN HEALTH

Thus, sunlight is a major environmental factor responsible for skin changes and avoidance of UV exposure is an important strategy to protect skin. However, other parameters such as genetic makeup or nutrition are also relevant for the maintenance of skin function and health. An adequate supply to the skin of nutrients is required for proper function and supplementation with selected dietary components may be suitable to support therapeutic intervention (11).

Consumption of certain plants or fish oils providing n-3 fatty acids modulates the arachidonic cascade and is of use in the treatment of inflammatory skin disorders. Diets rich in n-3 polyunsaturated fatty acids improve psoriasis symptoms while inflammatory processes are suppressed (12). A well-balanced diet sufficient in proteins, lipids, carbohydrates, vitamins and minerals is important for skin wound healing.

Much attention has been paid to adequately supplying the skin with dietary antioxidants including minerals such as Se, Mn, Cu and Zn, and the antioxidant vitamins C and E (13). Minerals are essential constituents of antioxidant enzymes. Vitamin C is one of the most powerful, least toxic natural antioxidants and is present in high concentrations in many tissues. It is required as a cofactor in the hydroxylation of proline residues in collagen. Vitamin C is essential for the maintenance of normal connective tissue as well as for wound healing. The term vitamin E comprises all tocols and tocotrienol derivatives which exhibit the biological activity of α-tocopherol (14). This group of compounds is highly lipophilic, operative in membranes or lipoproteins. Their most important antioxidant function appears to be the inhibition of lipid peroxidation, scavenging lipid peroxyl radicals to yield lipid hydroperoxides and a tocopheroxyl radical. Human and animal studies have shown that vitamin E and vitamin C provide UV-protection when the compounds are applied topically and systemically (15, 16). Further important dietary constituents with antioxidant activity and skin-protecting properties include the group carotenoids (17, 18).

3. CAROTENOIDS IN SKIN PROTECTION

Carotenoids have been applied for systemic photoprotection for several decades. They are used in the treatment of photosensitivity disorders, mainly porphyrias, and in healthy people as oral protectants against skin damage following sun exposure. Studies related to the latter topic are mainly linked to the prevention of primary skin responses such as sunburn (erythema solare). The prevention of UV-induced damage by carotenoids has also been investigated using biomarkers of photooxidative modifications of macromolecules like oxidized DNA bases, thymine dimers or protein carbonyls, both *in vitro* and *in vivo*. Furthermore, it should be stressed that some experimental studies in animals and cell culture provide evidence that carotenoids may be useful agents in the prevention of skin cancer (19). However, this has not been confirmed by epidemiological or interventional studies (20, 21).

3.1 ERYTHROPOIETIC PROTOPORPHYRIA

ß-carotene and other carotenoids, including lycopene, are successfully applied to ameliorate secondary effects of erythropoietic protoporphyria (EPP). EPP is a genetic disorder affecting porphyrin synthesis. As a consequence of ferrochelatase deficiency, the heme precursor protoporphyrin IX accumulates; this porphyrin is a strong photosensitizing agent. Upon light exposure photooxidative reactions are initiated, finally leading to skin damage; singlet molecular oxygen and electronically excited triplet states of suitable sensitizers are involved in the pathogenesis of EPP. A percentage of the patients suffering from EPP respond positively to treatment with high doses of carotenoids (up to 180 mg ß-carotene/d for several months); the symptoms following photosensitation are ameliorated (22-24). Quenching of singlet molecular oxygen via energy transfer between carotenoids and the electronically excited molecule are suggested to be the mechanism of protection.

3.2 β-CAROTENE IN PHOTOPROTECTION

ß-carotene is the most prominent carotenoid and commonly used as a component of dietary supplements. Specifically designed supplements with ß-carotene as a major constituent are sold as so-called oral sun protectants. Data from human studies on the UV-protective effects of orally applied ß-carotene in healthy people are contradictory. In a number of studies a moderate protection against UV-induced erythema has been found while no photoprotection was found in others. The study designs were different with respect to duration, dose, and methods used for the determination of photoprotection. It has been suggested that the efficacy of ß-carotene supplementation depends on the duration of treatment and on the dose. In studies where protection was found, treatment with carotenoids was for at least 10 weeks, and the dose was higher than 20 mg of carotenoids per day (23, 25-27). In studies reporting no protective effects carotenoids were applied for only 3-8 weeks (28, 29). Based on these findings it has been concluded that the application of moderate doses of ß-carotene alone is not sufficient to obtain sustained photoprotection (29).

Concerns about the safety of ß-carotene when applied in high doses raised a discussion on suitable dose levels for photoprotection (30). In two intervention studies where ß-carotene was applied for several years at doses of 20 and 30 mg per day, alone or in combination with α-tocopherol or retinol (31, 32), an increased incidence for lung cancer of about 20% was found in individuals at high risk for cancer (33).

As a consequence, ß-carotene was partially substituted by other carotenoids to obtain a combined carotenoid supplement and the photoprotective effects of such a combination were investigated (34). A mixture consisting of ß-carotene, lutein and lycopene (8 mg each/d) exhibited photoprotective effects comparable to those of a high dose of ß-carotene (24 mg/d) when applied for a period of 12 weeks. Using an antioxidant mixture providing 6 mg of ß-carotene and 6 mg of lycopene per day (with additional 10 mg RRR-α-tocopherol and 75 µg selenium), protection against UV-induced skin damage was achieved in humans (35). Intervention for a period of 7 weeks resulted in elevation of the actinic erythema threshold and diminished UV-induced erythema.

4. LYCOPENE IN SKIN PROTECTION

Due particularly to its chemical and biological properties, lycopene is an interesting dietary carotenoid with possible photoprotecting activity. Lycopene is a very unpolar non-provitamin A carotenoid present in human blood and tissues (36). It is the colorant of tomatoes, water melon and the pink grapefruit. In contrast to most of the other carotenoids there is only one major source of lycopene in the human diet (37). More than 80% of lycopene consumed in the United States is derived from tomato products. Processing of food helps to release lycopene from the food matrix, thus improving accessibility of the lipophilic compound for the formation of lipid micelles together with dietary lipids and bile acids (38). Cooking and food processing enhance the bioavailability of carotenoids; e.g. lycopene uptake is higher after ingestion of processed tomatoes (tomato paste) as compared to fresh tomatoes (39).

Among carotenoids lycopene is the most efficient singlet oxygen quencher (40). The interaction of carotenoids with $^1O_2$ depends largely on physical quenching which involves direct energy transfer between both molecules. The energy of singlet molecular oxygen is transferred to the carotenoid molecule to yield ground state oxygen and a triplet excited carotene. Instead of further chemical reactions, the carotenoid returns to ground state dissipating its energy by interaction with the surrounding solvent.

Lycopene also exhibits antioxidant properties *in vivo* (41). After consumption of lycopene-rich diets lycopene levels were increased in blood and the total antioxidant potential in serum was elevated.

Apart from its antioxidant activity other biochemical properties have also been attributed to lycopene which may be relevant in context with its preventing properties (42). Effects on the proliferation of cancer cells have been associated with the inhibition of cell cycle progression from the G0/G1 to the S phase. The compound also interferes with IGF-1 dependent pathways and induces detoxifying phase II enzymes.

4.1 LYCOPENE IN PHOTOPROTECTION

Studies in cell culture and animals have shown that lycopene prevents UV-induced photodamage. UVB-induced formation of malondialdehyde, a biomarker of lipid peroxidation, was lowered in human fibroblasts in the presence of carotenoids (43). Based on the levels needed for optimal protection, lycopene was a better antioxidant than ß-carotene and lutein. At higher levels all of the investigated carotenoids exhibited prooxidant effects. Photoprotection was also investigated in the exposure of human skin fibroblasts to UVA (44). No protection against UVA-induced expression of metalloproteinase 1 and heme-oxygenase 1 was found with lycopene and ß-carotene alone. However, in the presence of vitamin E the stability of both carotenoids in cell culture was improved and metalloproteinase 1 expression was suppressed. Topically applied, lycopene contributes to the prevention of UVB-induced photodamage (45). In a mouse, model application of lycopene inhibited UVB-induced ornithine decarboxylase and myeloperoxidase activity.

Human studies on the photoprotective effects of lycopene after systemic application are scarce. For most of the investigations, lycopene-rich products derived from tomatoes have been used as a source of the carotenoid.

The results described in the following paragraphs have been elaborated in our laboratory and describe photoprotective effects of dietary lycopene from various sources (46-48). The design was comparable in all of the studies. Readout for photoprotection was the prevention of erythema (reddening of the skin) after UV-irradiation. All volunteers that participated in the studies were of skin type II, according to the Fitzpatrick classification for sun-reactive skin types. The individual sensitivity towards erythematogenic UV exposure is characterized by the minimal erythemal dose (MED) which is defined as the lowest dose of UV radiation that will produce a detectable erythema 24 h after exposure. MED for each individual was determined prior to the study. Inclusion criteria were healthy condition, body mass index (BMI) of 18 – 25 kg/m^2, no pregnancy or lactation, no supplementation with vitamins, and no medication during the study. For intervention, the volunteers consumed lycopene from different sources for a period of 10-12 weeks.

At the beginning, during, and at the end of the study selected skin areas were irradiated with 1.25-fold the MED using a blue-light solar simulator and skin color was evaluated before and 24h after irradiation. Skin color was determined by chromametry using the three-dimensional color system where L-values are a parameter for lightness of skin and b-values (blue/yellow-axis) are indicative for pigmentation. Chromametry a-values (red/green-axis) determine redness of the skin and are used to evaluate the extent of reddening after irradiation. Subtracting the a-value before irradiation (individual basal redness of the skin) from the a-value determined after irradiation gives a Δ-a value. Decreasing Δ-a values during the study indicate protection against UV-induced erythema; Δ-a values at the beginning of the study were set at 100% and the others calculated as the percentage of basal numbers. At time points of UV exposure blood samples were taken and analyzed for lycopene and other carotenoids. Levels of total carotenoids in the skin were measured at the same time points by means of reflection spectroscopy (49).

4.2 LYCOPENE SUPPLEMENTS

The following lycopene supplements and a lycopene enriched drink were ingested over a period of 12 weeks to investigate photoprotective effects (46):

1. Lycopene soft gel capsules (Lyc-o-Mato®, LycoRed, Natural Prod. Industr. Ltd., Beer-Sheva, Israel) which contained a tomato extract; assigned as lycopene supplement. Two capsules were ingested per day mounting to a daily dose of 9.8 mg lycopene and 0.4 mg ß-carotene.
2. A lycopene-containing drink which was prepared from tomato extract (Lyc-o-Guard-Drink, LycoRed, Israel). Volunteers ingested 2 x 250 ml of the drink providing a total dose of 8.1 mg of lycopene and 0.4 mg of ß-carotene per day (lycopene drink).
3. Synthetic lycopene: volunteers ingested two hard shell capsules per day which contained synthetic lycopene encapsuled as beadlets; the dose was 10.2 mg/day.

The difference between chromametry a-values after and before irradiation (Δ a-value) were taken as a measure for UV-response of the skin and the results are shown in Fig.1.

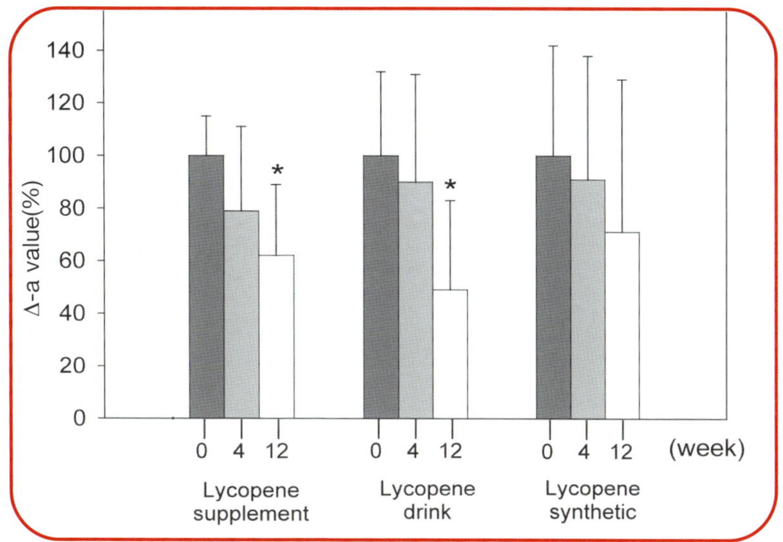

Fig. 1:Δ a-values of skin of volunteers (% baseline) on day 0, week 4 and week 12 after supplementation with different lycopene supplements (for details see text).*Significantly different from week 0 ($p < 0.05$)

A decrease in Δ a-values was found in all three groups indicating photoprotection. The change was statistically significant only after 12 weeks of supplementation with the lycopene supplement and the lycopene drink. No statistically significant photoprotection was found with the intake of synthetic lycopene. The dose was comparable between groups. However, tomato-based products contain a number of other constituents including further carotenoids such as ß-carotene, phytofluene and phytoene which may well contribute to photoprotection too.
After 4 weeks of supplementation, lycopene serum levels were increased in all groups reaching values between 0.55 and 0.84 nmol/ml which is about 2-fold the basal level. Between weeks 4 and 12 lycopene levels barely increased any further. In contrast to the serum, carotenoid skin levels were less affected; increases were measured in all study groups. At the end of the study, skin levels were elevated 1.2 to 1.4-fold compared to baseline.

4.3 PHOTOPROTECTIVE EFFECTS OF LYCOPENE-RICH DIETARY ITEMS

In order to investigate photoprotective effects provided by lycopene-rich dietary items carrot juice and tomato paste were used as lycopene sources (47, 48). The carrot juice (Fruchtsaft Bayer & Co, Ditzingen, Germany) was prepared from the variety "Nutrired" which is rich in lycopene. Volunteers consumed 2 x 200 ml of juice providing a total dose of 10 mg of lycopene and 5.1 mg of ß-carotene per day; duration of the study was 12 weeks. The tomato paste group consumed 40 g of tomato paste once a day together with 10 g of olive oil in order to improve carotenoid uptake. With the tomato paste 16 mg lycopene were ingested per day; duration of the study was 10 weeks.
A pronounced photoprotective effect was determined in the group that consumed the lycopene-rich carrot juice (Fig.2).

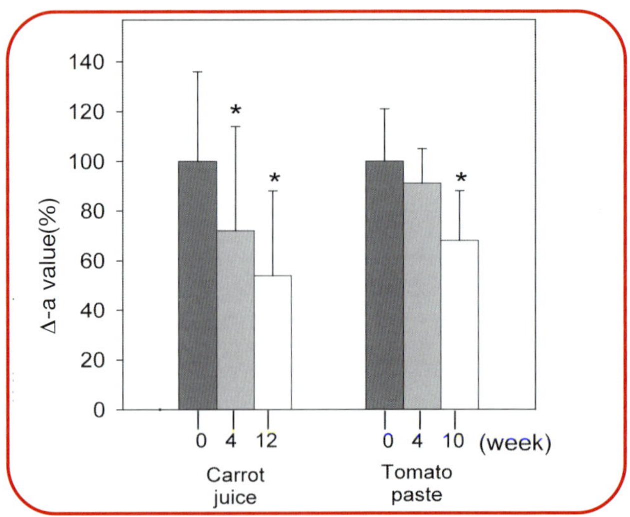

Fig. 2: Δ a-values of skin of volunteers (% baseline) on day 0, week 4 and week 10/12 after ingestion of lycopene from dietary sources.*Significantly different from week 0 ($p < 0.05$)

Δ a-values were significantly lower on week 4 and week 12 compared to baseline. At the end of the study the decrease was about 45%. Following the ingestion of tomato paste, a decrease in the Δ a-values from week 0 to week 4 and week 10 was determined. The difference was most pronounced and statistically significant on week 10. In comparison to baseline the Δ a-value was lowered by about 40%. Lycopene serum levels increased in the carrot juice group about 1.5-fold from 0.36 µM at baseline to 0.58 µM after 12 weeks of intervention. In the tomato paste group the mean lycopene level at baseline was 0.37µM rising to 0.72 µM at week 10 of the study. The differences observed between the groups may be due to differences in bioavailability of lycopene from the various sources but may also be related to interindividual variations with respect to lycopene uptake and/or distribution and metabolism.
The studies demonstrate that lycopene-rich products are suitable for endogenous photoprotection in the human skin.

5. EFFECTS OF CAROTENOIDS ON SKIN STRUCTURE AND TEXTURE

According to the studies mentioned above, carotenoids including lycopene are suitable protectants against UV-induced erythema. However, dietary constituents may also influence skin parameters including texture, colour, moisture, and other physiological properties. As with any other tissue, skin requires an optimal supply of nutritive compounds including macronutrients such as lipids, amino acids or carbohydrates and micronutrients like carotenoids, vitamins and essential minerals (11). Skin structure and function are affected by endogenous and environmental factors with either beneficial or adverse effects on skin health. However, *in vivo* data on the intake of micronutrients, especially carotenoids and their effects on skin appearance, are scarce.

A recent study provided evidence that long-term supplementation with a mixture of antioxidants containing lycopene and ß-carotene, 6 and 4.8 mg per day, respectively, as well as α-tocopherol (10 mg/day) and selenium (75 µg/day) affects parameters of skin physiology (50). Applying ultrasound measurements (B-Scan) it was shown that skin density and thickness improved during supplementation. Compared to the basal value, skin density was increased about 7% and skin thickness about 15%, after 6 and 12 weeks of supplementation.
During the study, skin surface parameters were determined using the SELS method. The “surface evaluation of living skin” (SELS) is based on the evaluation of an image of living skin taken under certain illumination; the picture is electronically processed for quantitative analyses. Appearance of the skin surface is described by four different parameters: “roughness”, “scaling”, “smoothness” and “wrinkling”.

Upon supplementation with the antioxidant mixture the SELS parameters scaling and roughness were improved. After 12 weeks of intervention roughness was decreased by about 30% and scaling by about 45% compared to the starting level; both changes were statistically significant. Smoothness and wrinkling were not affected by treatment.

During the study, at time points 0, 6 , and 12 weeks, lycopene, ß-carotene, lutein, zeaxanthin, α-carotene, cryptoxanthin, phytoene and phytofluene as well as α-tocopherol, γ-tocopherol, and retinol were analyzed in blood samples of the volunteers. At baseline the levels of the micronutrients were within the range of variance reported in the literature. After 12 weeks of supplementation, lycopene and ß-carotene levels increased to yield final concentrations of 0.88 and 1.33 nmol/ml, respectively. Both compounds were present in the supplement. Increases in phytoene and phytofluene were also measured. Both carotenoids are precursors of lycopene and ß-carotene and are present in carotenoid supplements which contain fruit or vegetable oleoresins. Tocopherol levels were not significantly increased.

This study demonstrates that supplementing a mixture of antioxidants improves skin physiology and can provide cosmetic effects. It remains unclear which of the compounds is a major contributor to effects and which mechanisms underly the improvement of skin conditions. However, carotenoids (especially lycopene) may act as antioxidants defending against external challenge of reactive oxygen species and contributing to skin health by improving cellular functions via non-antioxidant pathways.

6. CONCLUSION

Dietary micronutrients including the carotenoid lycopene are useful in the protection against excess light. Human intervention studies demonstrate that lycopene is a suitable endogenous photoprotectant. It should be noted that endogenous protection in terms of sun protection factor may be low or even marginal but the cumulative effect receives increasing attention. Lifelong inadvertent exposure is important (51). Improvement of the basal defense systems contributes to life-long protection against UV-dependent skin damage. Claims on cosmetic effects of micronutrients have been made, and an array of natural compounds is used in topically applied cosmetic products. The field of cosmeceuticals is in its developing stages. Providing endogenous nutrients for optimum skin health and care is an interesting new aspect. However, such concept lacks suitable data from nutrition research and only a few examples demonstrate the efficacy of dietary intervention to improve skin physiology.

REFERENCES :

1. Bruls, W. A., Slaper, H., van der Leun, J. C. & Berrens, L. (1984) Transmission of human epidermis and stratum corneum as a function of thickness in the ultraviolet and visible wavelengths. Photochem. Photobiol. 40: 485-494.
2. Hoffmann, K., Kaspar, K., Altmeyer, P. & Gambichler, T. (2000) UVtransmission measurements of small skin specimens with special quartz cuvettes.Dermatology 201: 307-311.
3. Krutmann, J. (2000) Ultraviolet A radiation-induced biological effects inhuman skin: relevance for photoaging and photodermatosis. J. Dermatol. Sci. 23 Suppl 1:S22-S26.
4. Schieke, S., Stege, H., Kurten, V., Grether-Beck, S., Sies, H. & Krutmann,J. (2002) Infrared-A radiation-induced matrix metalloproteinase 1 expression is mediated through extracellular signal-regulated kinase 1/2 activation in human dermal fibroblasts. J. Invest Dermatol. 119: 1323-1329.
5. Girotti, A. W. (2001) Lipid photooxidative damage in biological membranes: reaction mechanisms, cytotoxic consequences, and defense strategies. In:Sun Protection in Man (Giacomoni, P. U. ed.), pp. 231-250. Elsevier, Amsterdam.
6. Pinnell, S. R. (2003) Cutaneous photodamage, oxidative stress, and topical antioxidant protection. J. Am. Acad. Dermatol. 48: 1-19.
7. Ravanat, J.-L., Douki, T. & Cadet, J. (2001) UV damage to nucleic acid components. In: Sun Protection in Man (Giacomoni, P. U. ed.), pp. 207-230. Elsevier, Amsterdam.
8. Wenk, J., Brenneisen, P., Meewes, C., Wlaschek, M., Peters, T.,Blaudschun, R., Ma, W., Kuhr, L., Schneider, L. & Scharffetter-Kochanek, K. (2001) UV-induced oxidative stress and photoaging. Curr. Probl. Dermatol. 29: 83-94.
9. Davies, M. J. (2003) Singlet oxygen-mediated damage to proteins and its consequences. Biochem. Biophys. Res. Commun. 305: 761-770.
10. Dummer, R. & Maier, T. (2002) UV protection and skin cancer. In: Cancers of the Skin (Dumer, R., Nestle, F. O. & Burg, G. eds.), pp. 7-12. Springer, Heidelberg.
11. Boelsma, E., van de Vijver, L. P., Goldbohm, R. A., Klopping-Ketelaars, I. A., Hendriks, H. F. & Roza, L. (2003) Human skin condition and its associations with nutrient concentrations in serum and diet. Am. J. Clin. Nutr. 77: 348-355.
12. Boelsma, E., Hendriks, H. F. & Roza, L. (2001) Nutritional skin care:health effects of micronutrients and fatty acids. Am. J. Clin. Nutr. 73: 853-864.
13. Mukhtar, H. (2003) Eat plenty of green leafy vegetables for photoprotection: emerging evidence. J. Invest Dermatol. 121: viii.
14. Traber, M. G. & Sies, H. (1996) Vitamin E in humans: demand and delivery. Annu. Rev. Nutr. 16: 321-347.
15. Sies, H. & Stahl, W. (2004) Nutritional protection against skin damage from sunlight. Annu. Rev. Nutr. 24: 173-200.
16. F'guyer, S., Afaq, F. & Mukhtar, H. (2003) Photochemoprevention of skin cancer by botanical agents. Photodermatol. Photoimmunol. Photomed. 19: 56-72.
17. Stahl, W. & Sies, H. (2004) Carotenoids in systemic protection against sunburn. In: Carotenoids in Health and Disease (Krinsky, N. I., Mayne, S. T. & Sies, H. eds.), pp. 491-502. Marcel Dekker, New York.
18. Krinsky, N. I. & Johnson, E. J. (2005) Carotenoid actions and their relation to health and disease. Mol. Aspects Med. 26: 459-516.

19. Kune, G. A., Bannerman, S., Field, B., Watson, L. F., Cleland, H., Merenstein, D. & Vitetta, L. (1992) Diet, alcohol, smoking, serum beta-carotene, and vitamin A in male nonmelanocytic skin cancer patients and controls. Nutr. Cancer 18: 237-244.
20. Anstey, A. V. (2002) Systemic photoprotection with alpha-tocopherol (vitamin E) and beta-carotene. Clin. Exp. Dermatol. 27: 170-176.
21. Baron, J. A., Bertram, J. S., Britton, G., Buiatti, E., De Flora, S., Feron, V. J., Gerber, M., Greenberg, E. R., Kavlock, R. J. et al. (1998) IARC Handbooks of cancer prevention: Carotenoids vol 2. IARC, Lyon.
22. Fritsch, C., Bolsen, K., Ruzicka, T. & Goerz, G. (1997) Congenital erythropoietic porphyria. J. Am. Acad. Dermatol. 36: 594-610.
23. Mathews-Roth, M. M., Pathak, M. A., Parrish, J. A., Fitzpatrick, T. B., Kass, E. H., Toda, K. & Clemens, W. (1972) A clinical trial of the effects of oral betacarotene on the responses of human skin to solar radiation. J. Invest. Dermatol. 59: 349-353.
24. von Laar, J., Stahl, W., Bolsen, K., Goerz, G. & Sies, H. (1996) β-carotene serum levels in patients with erythropoietic protoporphyria on treatment with the synthetic all-trans isomer or a natural isomer mixture of β-carotene. J. Photochem.Photobiol. B:Biol. 33: 157-162.
25. Gollnick, H. P. M., Hopfenmüller, W., Hemmes, C., Chun, S. C., Schmid, C., Sundermeier, K. & Biesalski, H. K. (1996) Systemic beta carotene plus topical UVsunscreen are an optimal protection against harmful effects of natural UV-sunlight: results of the Berlin-Eilath study. Eur. J. Dermatol. 6: 200-205.
26. Lee, J., Jiang, S., Levine, N. & Watson, R. R. (2000) Carotenoid supplementation reduces erythema in human skin after simulated solar radiation exposure. Proc. Soc. Exp. Biol. Med. 223: 170-174.
27. Stahl, W., Heinrich, U., Jungmann, H., Sies, H. & Tronnier, H. (2000) Carotenoids and carotenoids plus vitamin E protect against ultraviolet light-induced erythema in humans. Am. J. Clin. Nutr. 71: 795-798.
28. Garmyn, M., Ribaya-Mercado, J. D., Russell, R. M., Bhawan, J. & Gilchrest, B. A. (1995) Effect of beta-carotene supplementation on the human sunburn reaction. Exp. Dermatol. 4: 104-111.
29. McArdle, F., Rhodes, L. E., Parslew, R. A., Close, G. L., Jack, C. I., Friedmann, P. S. & Jackson, M. J. (2004) Effects of oral vitamin E and beta-carotene supplementation on ultraviolet radiation-induced oxidative stress in human skin. Am. J. Clin. Nutr. 80: 1270-1275.
30. Biesalski, H. K. & Obermüller-Jevic, U. C. (2001) UV light, beta-carotene and human skin-beneficial and potentially harmful effects. Arch. Biochem. Biophys. 389: 1-6.
31. Omenn, G. S., Goodman, G. E., Thornquist, M. D., Balmes, J., Cullen, M. R., Glass, A., Keogh, J. P., Meyskens, F. L., Valanis, B. et al. (1996) Risk factors for lung cancer and for intervention effects in CARET, the beta-carotene and retinol efficacy trial. J. Natl. Cancer Inst. 88: 1550-1559.
32. Albanes, D., Heinonen, O. P., Taylor, P. R., Virtamo, J., Edwards, B. K., Rautalahti, M., Hartman, A. M., Palmgren, J., Freedman, L. S. et al. (1996) Alpha-Tocopherol and beta-carotene supplements and lung cancer incidence in the alphatocopherol, beta-carotene cancer prevention study: effects of base-line characteristics and study compliance. J. Natl. Cancer Inst. 88: 1560-1570.
33. The ATBC-Study Group (1994) The effect of vitamin E and beta carotene on the incidence of lung cancer and other cancers in male smokers. N. Engl. J. Med. 330: 1029-1035.

34. Heinrich, U., Gartner, C., Wiebusch, M., Eichler, O., Sies, H., Tronnier, H. & Stahl, W. (2003) Supplementation with beta-carotene or a similar amount of mixed carotenoids protects humans from UV-induced erythema. J. Nutr. 133: 98-101.
35. Cesarini, J. P., Michel, L., Maurette, J. M., Adhoute, H. & Bejot, M. (2003) Immediate effects of UV radiation on the skin: modification by an antioxidant complex containing carotenoids. Photodermatol. Photoimmunol. Photomed. 19: 182-189.
36. Stahl, W. & Sies, H. (1996) Lycopene: a biologically important carotenoid for humans? Arch. Biochem. Biophys. 336: 1-9.
37. Canene-Adams, K., Campbell, J. K., Zaripheh, S., Jeffery, E. H., Erdman, J. W., Jr. (2005). The tomato as a functional food. J. Nutr. 135:1226-30.
38. Williams, A. W., Boileau, T. W. M. & Erdman, J. W. (1998) Factors influencing the uptake and absorption of carotenoids. Proc. Soc. Exp. Biol. Med. 218: 106-108.
39. Gärtner, C., Stahl, W. & Sies, H. (1997) Lycopene is more bioavailable from tomato paste than from fresh tomatoes. Am. J. Clin. Nutr. 66: 116-122.
40. Di Mascio, P., Kaiser, S. & Sies, H. (1989) Lycopene as the most efficient biological carotenoid singlet oxygen quencher. Arch. Biochem. Biophys. 274: 532-538.
41. Rao, A. V. (2004) Processed tomato products as a source of dietary lycopene: bioavailability and antioxidant properties. Can. J. Diet. Pract. Res. 65: 161-165.
42. Sharoni, Y., Danilenko, M., Levy, J. & Stahl, W. (2004) Anticancer activity of carotenoids: from human studies to cellular processes and gene regulation. In:Carotenoids in Health and Disease (Krinsky, N. I., Mayne, S. T. & Sies, H. eds.), pp.165-196. Marcel Dekker, New York.
43. Eichler, O., Sies, H. & Stahl, W. (2002) Divergent optimum levels of lycopene, beta-carotene and lutein protecting against UVB irradiation in human fibroblasts. Photochem. Photobiol. 75: 503-506.
44. Offord, E. A., Gautier, J. C., Avanti, O., Scaletta, C., Runge, F., Kramer, K. & Applegate, L. A. (2002) Photoprotective potential of lycopene, beta-carotene, vitamin E, vitamin C and carnosic acid in UVA-irradiated human skin fibroblasts. Free Radic. Biol. Med. 32: 1293-1303.
45. Fazekas, Z., Gao, D., Saladi, R. N., Lu, Y., Lebwohl, M. & Wei, H. (2003) Protective effects of lycopene against ultraviolet B-induced photodamage. Nutr. Cancer 47: 181-187.
46. Aust, O., Stahl, W., Sies, H., Tronnier, H. & Heinrich, U. (2005) Supplementation with tomato-based products increases lycopene, phytofluene, and phytoene levels in human serum and protects against UV-light-induced erythema. Int. J. Vitam. Nutr. Res. 75: 54-60.
47. Stahl, W., Heinrich, U., Wiseman, S., Eichler, O., Sies, H. & Tronnier, H. (2001) Dietary tomato paste protects against ultraviolet light-induced erythema in humans. J. Nutr. 131: 1449-1451.
48. Stahl, W., Heinrich, U., Aust, O., Tronnier, H. & Sies, H. (2006) Lycopene-rich products and dietary photoprotection. Photochem. Photobiol. Sci. in press
49. Stahl, W., Heinrich, U., Jungmann, H., von Laar, J., Schietzel, M., Sies, H. & Tronnier, H. (1998) Increased dermal carotenoid levels assessed by noninvasive reflection spectrophotometry correlate with serum levels in women ingesting Betatene. J. Nutr. 128: 903-907.
50. Heinrich, U., Tronnier, H., Stahl, W., Bejot, M. & Maurette, J. M. (2006) Antioxidant supplements improve parameters related to skin structure in humans. Skin Pharmacol. Physiol. in press
51. Godar, D. E., Urbach, F., Gasparro, F. P. & van der Leun, J. C. (2003) UV doses of young adults. Photochem. Photobiol. 77: 453-457.

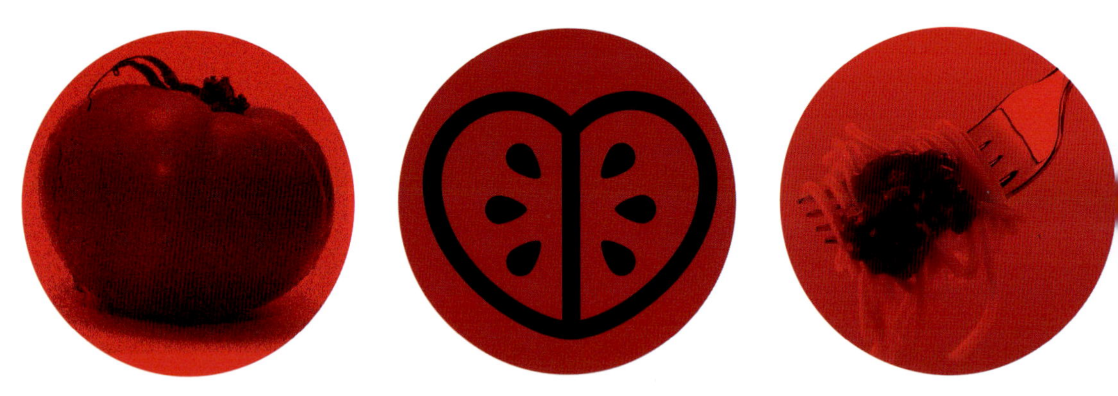

Lycocard: a promising new project

EU Commission funded within the Sixth Research Framework Programme. Role of lycopene for the prevention of cardiovascular diseases

Volker Böhm,
Institute of Nutrition,
Friedrich Schiller University
Jena, Germany

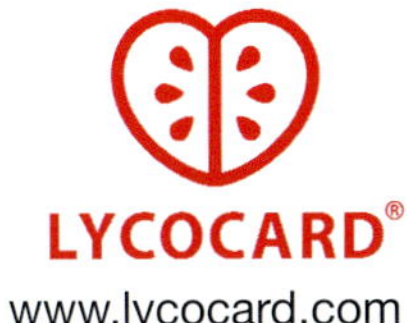

www.lycocard.com

Introduction

Cardiovascular diseases, along with cancer, are the main mortality causes in Europe and other developed countries. Lycopene is a plant pigment found in high concentration in red fruits, especially tomatoes – Europe's second-most important crop. Strong correlative evidence suggests that lycopene may provide important protection against cardiovascular diseases and cancer. However, these two aspects – lycopene content of tomatoes and lycopene's beneficial effects – have not been sufficiently linked because research has lacked a "total food chain" approach. The missing links in the chain are the development of healthy new foods and nutritional guidelines. There are also many details regarding bioavailability, metabolism, and molecular mechanisms of lycopene biological activities that are still unknown. LYCOCARD, an Integrated Project (6th Research Framework Programme) that started in April 2006, running for five years with a budget of 5.2 million euros, will investigate the role of lycopene in reducing the risk of cardiovascular diseases, adopting a "total food chain" approach by addressing each link in a "farm to fork" approach.

Fifteen partners from six European countries form LYCOCARD's multidisciplinary, intersectorial consortium of scientists, technologists, industrial bodies, scientific publishers and patient organisations giving it the critical mass to achieve these ambitious aims. Specifically, LYCOCARD will clarify the following points: effects of technological processing on lycopene, interactions between different food ingredients, molecular aspects of absorption and metabolism of lycopene, and biological effects of lycopene isomers and lycopene metabolites. This information will lead to improved nutritional guidelines and healthy new foods based on tomatoes. These novel dietary guidelines will help consumers select specific diets to prevent and minimise their disease risk. LYCOCARD will thus improve the health of consumers in Europe and worldwide while helping to reduce the costs of health systems, simultaneously and significantly advancing the state of the art. In addition, the position of the European (and worldwide) food industry will be strengthened by increasing the demand for health-related tomato products.

STATE OF THE ART

The risk factors that predispose one to cardiovascular diseases have been identified by means of several studies in well-defined population groups (1, 2). Among the most important "cardiovascular risk factors" are cigarette smoking and serum cholesterol levels. Smoking has been reported to increase atherosclerotic diseases by about 50% and at least doubles the incidence of coronary artery disease. Moreover, considerable evidence supports the direct relation between cardiovascular diseases and increased levels of serum low-density lipoprotein (LDL) cholesterol. There is now a scientific consensus that atherosclerosis represents a state of increased oxidative stress characterised by lipid and protein oxidation in the vascular wall. One initial step leading to the development of atherosclerosis might be the oxidation of unsaturated lipids in the LDL particles (3, 4). Human LDL particles are heterogeneous in nature, and the smaller and denser particles are more prone to oxidation. There is much debate about the antioxidant content of these particles, and carotenoids, mainly lycopene, may play a key role in protecting LDL particles. In addition to LDL oxidation, other oxidative events are involved in vascular diseases. These include the production of reactive oxygen and nitrogen species by vascular cells, as well as oxidative modifications contributing to important clinical manifestations of coronary artery disease, such as endothelial dysfunction and plaque disruption. The contribution of antioxidants to cardiovascular diseases has been investigated to some degree; however, only scarce data are available about the specific effects of lycopene or tomato products (5-10).

Diet is believed to play a major role in the development of cardiovascular diseases. The gastric digestion of food containing oxidisable lipids and iron catalysts for peroxide decomposition (such as (met)myoglobin from muscle meat) can be accompanied by an extensive formation of potentially toxic lipid hydroperoxides which are implicated in the process of atherosclerosis. Much interest and research are focused on identifying ways to prevent cardiovascular diseases through dietary changes. Primarily, epidemiological studies as well as some *in vitro* and limited *in vivo* experiments support the hypothesis that carotenoids, including β-carotene and lycopene, may protect lipoproteins and vascular cells from oxidation. In particular, lycopene is known to be an efficient scavenger of reactive oxygen species, including singlet oxygen ($^1O_2$) and other excited species (11,12). Lycopene also reduces the amount of oxidative DNA damage in cell culture and in rats *in vivo* (13, 14). In addition, clinical studies demonstrated that a lycopene-rich diet protects against oxidative DNA damage in human leukocytes *in vitro* (15) and prostate tissue *in vivo* (16). Several findings suggest that the redox properties of carotenoid molecules can deeply influence cell growth, by affecting molecular pathways involved in cell proliferation and apoptosis. A variety of animal and cell-culture studies also supports a role for lycopene in cell growth. All together, these findings suggest that lycopene can modify cell growth of smooth muscle cells present in the atheroma.

Besides cardiovascular diseases, recent evidence points to carotenoids as effective antioxidants for inhibiting the development of degenerative diseases such as cancer, cataracts, etc. Intake of β-carotene has been inversely linked to incidence of lung cancer, and similar correlations have been shown between lutein and macular disease and between lycopene or tomato-based products and prostate cancer (17-19). However, lycopene, despite being the strongest singlet oxygen quencher as well as a potent antioxidant compared to other carotenoids, has rarely been tested in studies for its role in cardiovascular disease prevention. Although some papers (20-22) reported inverse correlation between incidence for degenerative diseases and the consumption of fruit and vegetable instead of correlations to single ingredients of these foods, there is only scarce scientific knowledge on the interactions between different food components regarding their protective potential. Important points of bioavailability of lycopene as well as molecular mechanisms of its protective effects are not yet completely investigated.

Lycopene is mainly contained in tomatoes, the second-most important vegetable in Europe (after potatoes) and in higher concentrations in processed tomato products like ketchup, tomato sauce/juice, as well as in red coloured fruits like water melon and guava. Accordingly, the main dietary source of lycopene in Europe and the US is processed tomato products. Tomatoes and tomato products have been under investigation for their protective effects on health for many years. However, the scientific reasons for their positive effects are not yet completely clear. Besides lycopene, which has been studied now for more than a decade, tomatoes contain other positive ingredients, including other carotenoids, ascorbic acid, tocopherols, folate, polyphenols, etc., whose interactions with lycopene have not yet been investigated in detail. Tomatoes have not been considered as an important source of folate in the diet, but due to their great consumption, the contribution of tomatoes to the total intake of folate might be relevant. A poor intake of folates in the diet has been associated with an increase of homocysteine level in human plasma, which is considered a risk factor in cardiovascular diseases. This brief review has shown that there is a wealth of information about development of cardiovascular diseases as well as good evidence that certain foods – such as tomatoes – are healthy. However, these two aspects are not sufficiently linked because research has lacked a "total food chain" approach. The missing link in the chain is the development of healthy new foods and nutritional guidelines that bring these two ends of the food chain together.

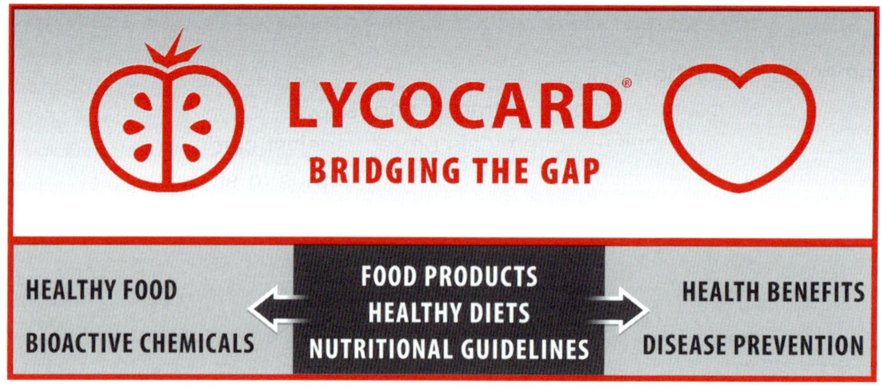

Figure 1: LYCOCARD s results will bridge the gap

LYCOCARD will significantly advance the state of the art because it will directly address missing links in the total chain of knowledge (Figure 1). Specifically, LYCOCARD will clarify the following points: effects of technological processes on lycopene, interactions between different food ingredients, major molecular aspects of absorption and metabolism of lycopene, and biological effects of lycopene isomers and lycopene metabolites. This information will lead to improved nutritional guidelines and healthy new foods. LYCOCARD will serve also as an example of how collaborative research and application can take up the "total food chain" and "farm-to-fork" approaches for future projects to increase the understanding of diet and health.

OBJECTIVES

Everyone knows that diet plays an important role in health. Whether from eating too much and developing obesity-related complications or eating too little and suffering the effects of starvation and malnutrition, the importance of foods to human health is certainly undeniable. What remains to a large extent unclear is exactly how many specific components of the foods we eat affect our health. What are those important compounds? What are the biochemical and physiological processes they interact with in affecting health? If a compound is shown to be good for us, can we find ways to increase the beneficial effects while minimising the risks? Can we create new foods and eating patterns that take advantage of these findings? These are some of the important questions that LYCOCARD will answer.

Specifically, LYCOCARD will investigate the role of lycopene in reducing the risk of cardiovascular diseases. Cardiovascular diseases, along with cancer, are the main mortality causes in Europe and other developed countries. Lycopene is a plant pigment found in high concentration in red fruits, especially tomatoes. Strong correlative evidence suggests that increased intake of lycopene may provide important protection against incidence of cardiovascular diseases and cancer. A search for "lycopene" on the web results in all sorts of sites providing recommendations on how to increase your lycopene intake via specific foods, tasty recipes, and of course various extracts and supplements. But exactly how lycopene and other associated chemicals protect against cardiovascular diseases remains unclear. The overall goal of LYCOCARD is thus to study the biochemical and physiological activity of lycopene and translate this understanding into development of new foods and dietary guidelines that improve the health and quality of life of European citizens. To achieve this ambitious goal, LYCOCARD has identified intermediate objectives in the following areas: Research, Development, Dissemination and Training.

RESEARCH OBJECTIVES

LYCOCARD will investigate different aspects of lycopene bioavailability by means of transporters, receptors and isomerisation. Another task will be to look for oxidative catabolism of lycopene after an antioxidant action or through chemical oxidations, in order to investigate the processes within the human body in detail. Physiologically relevant isomers and metabolites will be tested for their protective potential by using different *in vitro* and *ex vivo* methods. Modulation of various receptors and genes by these compounds is a further task. LYCOCARD will focus on their effects on endothelial cells and relevant signalling pathways regarding cardiovascular health. The two negative factors – cigarette smoke and cholesterol – will be investigated in *in vitro* and *ex vivo* models. The possible preventive roles of lycopene and lycopene isomers on the modifications induced by these toxic agents on redox status and on redox-sensitive molecular pathways as they affect processes of differentiation, proliferation and apoptosis of vascular cells will be investigated. All this research will constitute a significant advance beyond the current state of the art because it will move us away from simple correlations between particular foods and health benefits towards a detailed understanding of what specific aspects of these foods effect health benefits and how.

DEVELOPMENT OBJECTIVES

Research results will lead to more detailed knowledge of the protective effects of fruit and vegetables, mainly tomatoes and tomato products, and will allow the partners from the food industry to develop new foods with higher protective impact on cardiovascular health. The protective effects of these newly developed products will be tested. Finally, two patient organisations will use the results of the experiments to develop new dietary recommendations aimed at reducing (primary prevention) the incidence of cardiovascular diseases as well as provide guidelines for those people at risk. Because close links may exist among oxidative stress, inflammation, obesity, and cardiovascular disease, the effects of diets enriched with tomato products containing high levels of lycopene will be evaluated in obese patients.

DISSEMINATION OBJECTIVES

Two LYCOCARD partners are patient organisations that are experienced not only in the development of health guidelines, but also in the dissemination of knowledge about health research and development to the public. They do this through effective communication with stakeholders, for example medical associations and other patient advocacy groups. Consumers from all over Europe will thus be the primary beneficiaries of the LYCOCARD results. Not only will Europeans and people everywhere be able to enjoy a higher quality of life because of access to better information about the role of diet in health and availability of healthier foods, but also society will benefit because of reduced disease-related health-care costs.

In addition, the project will strengthen the position of the European and global food industry, mainly by enhancing opportunities for small and medium-sized enterprises (SMEs) in the agricultural and food processing industries. Specific health guidelines based on Europe's second-most important crop will strengthen agriculture, while development of tomato products by SMEs involved in the project will strengthen their competitiveness in the world market.

TRAINING OBJECTIVES

One of Europe's great opportunities and challenges is its diversity. This diversity will help in creating innovative solutions to our problems because of the range of backgrounds and outlooks brought to the table. This diversity also requires investment to build up capacity in certain regions and develop facility in cross-cultural and multi-disciplinary collaboration (strengthened network). LYCOCARD partners are excited about contributing to this process through training the next generation of highly skilled scientists, biotechnologists, and public health professionals. Our highly experienced lead scientists will be the mentors for a truly interdisciplinary experience for early-stage researchers. The lead scientists themselves will also build up their own and their institutions' capacities through strong collaborations within LYCOCARD's multi-cultural, multi-disciplinary team.

SUMMARY

- Overall goal: study of the biochemical and physiological activity of lycopene and development of new foods and dietary guidelines for improvement of health and quality of life

- Research objectives: understanding of physiological, biochemical and genetic roles of lycopene in protecting from cardiovascular diseases

- Development objectives: development of new foods high in health-promoting compounds and health guidelines and dietary recommendations

- Dissemination objectives: enhancement of health and quality of life through a better diet as well as enhancement of opportunities for SMEs

- Training objectives: training of a highly competent workforce of biotechnologists and scientists who are skilled in multidisciplinary, pan-European cooperation

REFERENCES:

1. W. B. Kannel, P. W. F. Wilson, An update on coronary risk factors, Med. Clin. North Am. 79 (1995) 951-971.
2. J. D. Neaton, D. Wentworth, Serum cholesterol, blood pressure, cigarette smoking, and death from coronary heart disease: overall findings and differences by age for 316.000 white men, Arch. Intern. Med. 152 (1992) 56-64.
3. R. A. Riemersma, Epidemiology and the role of antioxidants in preventing coronary heart disease: a brief overview, Proc. Nutr. Soc. 53 (1994) 59-65.
4. J. M. Gaziano et al., Supplementation with β-carotene in vivo and in vitro does not inhibit low density lipoprotein oxidation, Atherosclerosis 112 (1995) 187-195.
5. D. L. Morris, S. B. Kritchevsky, C. E. Davis, Serum carotenoids and coronary heart disease, J. Am. Med. Assoc. 272 (1994) 1439-1441.
6. [L. Kohlmeier et al., Lycopene and myocardial infarction risk in the EURAMIC study, Am. J. Epidemiol. 146 (1997) 618-626.
7. V. P. Palace, N. Khaper, Q. Qin, P. K. Singal, Antioxidant potentials of vitamin A and carotenoids and their relevance to heart disease, Free Radical Biol. Med. 26 (1999) 746-761.
8. R. Bilton, M. Gerber, P. Grolier, C. Leoni (eds), The White Book on antioxidants in tomatoes and tomato products and their health benefits, 2nd rev. edition 2001, CMITI Sarl Avignon, ISSN 1145-9565.
9. J. K. Willcox, G. L. Catignani, S. Lazarus, Tomatoes and cardiovascular health, Crit. Rev. Food Sci. Nutr. 43 (2003) 1-18.
10. D. P. Vivekananthan, M. S. Penn, S. K. Sapp, A. Hsu, Use of antioxidant vitamins for the prevention of cardiovascular disease: meta-analysis of randomized trials, Lancet 361 (2003) 2017-2023.
11. W. Stahl, B. Junghans, E. S. de Boer, E. S. Driomina, K. Briviba, H. Sies, Carotenoid mixtures protect multilamellar liposomes against oxidative damage: synergistic effects of lycopene and lutein, FEBS Lett. 427 (1998) 305-308.
12. A. A. Woodall, G. Britton, M. J. Jackson, Carotenoids and protection of phospholipids in solution or in liposomes against oxidation by peroxyl radicals: relationship between carotenoid structure and protective ability, Biochim. Biophys. Acta 1336 (1997) 575-586.
13. H. R. Matos, V. I. Capelozzi, O. F. Gomes, P. di Mascio, M. H. Medeiros, Lycopene inhibits DNA damage and liver necrosis in rats treated with ferric nitrilotriacetate, Arch. Biochem. Biophys. 396 (2001) 171-177.
14. H. R. Matos, P. di Mascio, M. H. Medeiros, Protective effect of lycopene on lipid peroxidation and oxidative DNA damage in cell cultures, Arch. Biochem. Biophys. 383 (2000) 56-59.
15. B. L. Pool-Zobel, A. Bub, H. M ller, I. Wollowsky, G. Rechkemmer, Consumption of vegetables reduces genetic damage in humans: first results of a human intervention trial with carotenoid-rich foods, Carcinogenesis 18 (1997) 1847-1850.
16. P. Bowen, I. Chen, M. Stacewicz-Sapuntzakis, C. Duncan, R. Sharifi, L. Ghosh, H. S. Kim, K. Christov-Tzelkov, R. van Breemen, Tomato sauce supplementation and prostate cancer: Lycopene accumulation and modulation of biomarkers of carcinogenesis, Exp. Biol. Med. 227 (2002) 886-893.
17. E. Giovannucci, E. B. Rimm, Y. Liu, M. J. Stampfer, W. C. Willet, A prospective study of tomato products, lycopene, and prostate cancer risk, J. Natl. Cancer Inst. 94 (2002) 391-398.

18. H. D. Sesso, J. E. Buring, E. P. Norkus, J. M. Gaziano, Plasma lycopene, other carotenoids, and retinol and the risk of cardiovascular disease in women, Am. J. Clin. Nutr. 79 (2004) 47-53.
19. D. A. Cooper, A. L. Elridge, J. C. Peters, Dietary carotenoids and certain cancers, heart disease, and age-related macular degeneration: A review of recent research, Nutr. Rev. 57 (1999) 201-214.
20. G. Block, B. Patterson, A. Subar, Fruit, vegetables, and cancer prevention: A review of the epidemiological evidence, Nutr. Cancer 18 (1992) 1-29.
21. S. Bradley, R. Shinton, Why is there an association between eating fruit and vegetables and a lower risk of stroke?, J. Human Nutr. Diet. 11 (1998) 363-372.
22. S. Franceschi, M. Parpinel, C. La Vecchia, A. Favero, R. Talamini, E. Negri, Role of different types of vegetables and fruit in the prevention of cancer of the colon, rectum, and breast, Epidemiol. 9 (1998) 338-341.

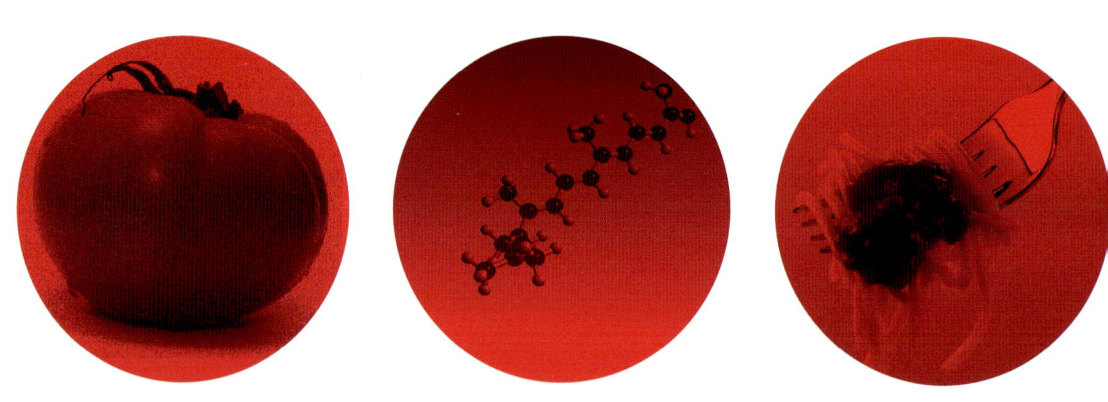

Lycopene and Human Health: Summary and Future Directions

Dr. A.V. Rao
Department of Nutritional Sciences
Faculty of Medicine
University of Toronto,
Ontario, Canada.

Introduction

In recent years there has been a dramatic increase in the availability of scientific and lay publications about the role of fruits and vegetables in human health. Over the last decade lycopene has been singled out as a significant factor and has received increasing amounts of attention on account of its potential role in the prevention of chronic diseases. From a few articles ten years ago to the several thousand reviewed papers and articles currently available. This book is a direct result of this growing interest and sets out to summarize the current state of knowledge in this area.

'*Tomatoes, Lycopene & Human Health*', provides, for the first time, comprehensive, up to date information on various aspects of tomato lycopene showing how we can protect our health simply through attention to our diet. Internationally recognized experts have contributed chapters to this book which will be of great interest to the scientific community, food related industries, government agencies and also consumers.

This book examines many aspects of tomato lycopene and human health including dietary guidelines recommending increased consumption of plant foods for the prevention of chronic diseases such as cancer, cardiovascular disease, osteoporosis and diabetes. Scientists are actively investigating the role of these nutrients in human health looking at the properties of phytochemicals, their occurrence, bioavailability, metabolism, mechanisms of action and how they can protect us. Much attention has been focused upon oxidative stress-induced cellular damage which is recognized as leading to the progression of chronic diseases. Antioxidants play an important role in stopping the harmful effects of oxidative stress. Phytochemicals including fat soluble carotenoids and water soluble polyphenols are important sources of plant antioxidants. Lycopene, a carotenoid antioxidant in tomatoes, tomato products and other fruits and vegetables is the focus of many recent studies. Tomatoes and tomato products are the main sources of lycopene in the human diet accounting for almost 80% of the total daily intake. Lycopene is a relatively stable compound able to survive heat processing and storage although some operations, such as freezing, reduce the lycopene content by 50%. Lycopene bioavailability is improved by heat processing and the presence of fat so cooking actually improves the nutritional value.

The antioxidant properties of lycopene in foods play a key role in human health. Lycopene is an important member of the carotenoid family and its antioxidant action allows it to remove damaging free radicals and quench 'singlet oxygen' species very effectively. Also, in the presence of vitamin C the used lycopene is converted back into its original form ready to act as an antioxidant again. Lycopene can also repair other oxidized carotenoids, such as zeaxanthin and lutein, involved in age-related blindness. In addition to its antioxidant properties, lycopene has other abilities which include improving communication between cancer cells, regulating cancer cell proliferation, performing immune surveillance and inhibiting liver metabolizing enzymes, cholesterol synthesis and inflammatory processes. Lycopene also interacts positively with vitamin D and other phytochemicals such as lutein. Oxidative damage of DNA is the main first step in the progression of cancers and lycopene has been shown to give protection from DNA oxidation in many human studies.

Chronic human diseases such as cancer, a multi-step process consisting of three main stages – initiation, promotion and progression. Lycopene can inhibit all three stages by blocking initiation, boosting detoxification and antioxidant enzymes and by stopping proliferation of the cancer cells.

CHEMOPREVENTION

Lycopene can now be referred to as a chemopreventive agent especially as new scientific evidence suggests the cancer preventing effects of lycopene may be the result of its synergistic interactions with other phytonutrients such as phytoene, phytofluenes and β-carotene found in tomatoes and tomato products. These positive interactions have led to the term 'combination prevention' of cancer. Tomatoes and tomato products are an effective blend of phytonutrients that play an important role in the prevention of cancers. Pre-clinical studies show that lycopene has potent *in vitro* and *in vivo* anti-tumour effects on prostate cancer cells suggesting potential preventive and therapeutic roles. The small numbers of patients in these clinical trials preclude any firm conclusions with regard to lycopenes use as a treatment though expanded research is certainly warranted.

CARDIOPROTECTION

Cardiovascular diseases (CVD) are a major public health problem, representing the most common cause of death in Europe and many other industrialized regions. There is growing evidence that a diet rich in carotenoids can protect against CVD. A review of epidemiological (population) studies provides convincing evidence in favor of a protective role for lycopene although further studies are needed for a fuller understanding. This book discusses a new, five year science project called Lycocard which is devoting substantial resources to studying the role of lycopene in the prevention of CVD. Lycocard is a multidisciplinary consortium of scientists, technologists, and patient organisations composed of fifteen partners from six European countries. Lycocard will examine the following points: effects of technological processing on lycopene, interactions between different food ingredients, molecular aspects of lycopene absorption and metabolism, and biological effects of lycopene isomers and metabolites. This information will lead to improved nutritional guidelines and healthy new tomato-based foods. Lycocard initiated the adoption of a "total food chain" approach by addressing each link in a "farm to fork" approach. This work began in April 2006 and is ongoing.

OSTEOPOROSIS

Another chronic disease currently being investigated, osteoporosis is a major metabolic bone disease that primarily affects women and men over the age of 50. One risk factor is oxidative stress caused by reactive oxygen species (ROS). Lycopene has been suggested in the prevention of osteoporosis in postmenopausal women based on epidemiological data. This is a new and very exciting area of study and could provoke serious dietary considerations for all people seeking to protect against this silent disease.

HYPERTENSION / MALE INFERTILITY

Hypertension is a significant factor in coronary heart diseases and oxidative stress is now recognized as a component of hypertension. The role of lycopene in preventing hypertension and the results of a recent clinical study are of great interest and discussed here in detail. Male infertility is an important condition also addressed in this book. Among the many causative factors, oxidative stress is considered one of the most important. Due to its composition, sperm is highly vulnerable to oxidative damage. A recently completed study shows how lycopene acting as an antioxidant can improve sperm quality.

SKIN CARE

A newer development is the application of lycopene in cosmeceutical products. UV-irradiation of human skin leads to photo-oxidative damage associated with adverse effects on skin health and appearance. Supplying the skin with micronutrients may produce a degree of photo-protection. Carotenoids are important components of the light-protecting system in plants and prevent UV damage in humans. The protective properties are due to the pronounced antioxidant effects of these compounds. Human intervention studies provide evidence that skin can be protected against UV-dependent lesions by administration of lycopene or more effectively by eating a lycopene-rich diet.

This book also reviews lycopene research in the food, pharmaceutical and nutrient supplement industries. Three areas are discussed that include the use of tomatoes with a high lycopene content, preventing lycopene loss during processing, and fortification and standardization of tomato products with natural tomato lycopene. It concludes by affirming that the health benefits of tomatoes and lycopene will have a significant impact on the tomato industry in the future.

RECOMMENDED DAILY INTAKE

Since humans do not synthesize lycopene, it has to be provided through diet. There is a general agreement among scientists that the average intake of lycopene is lower than required to obtain its beneficial effects. Since lycopene is not yet recognized as an essential nutrient, there is still no official recommended daily intake (RDI) level set by government regulatory agencies. However, based on reported studies, a level of 30-35 mg was initially suggested. More recent studies show that a daily intake of 7-8 mg is enough to maintain sufficient levels of lycopene to fight oxidative stress and prevent chronic diseases. However, in the case of patients with cancer and cardiovascular diseases, a higher level ranging from 35 –75mg per day may be required. There is still a big gap between the recommended daily intake of lycopene and the actual average daily intake around the world. We need to narrow or perhaps eliminate this gap by developing technology, education and providing innovative products.

FUTURE DIRECTIONS

Based on current information, there is convincing evidence to suggest that lycopene intake is related to the prevention of several chronic diseases. Although the initial interest in lycopene involved its role in cancer, cardiovascular disease is now also under consideration. At the same time scientists continue to investigate newer areas for the use of lycopene including in osteoporosis, hypertension, male infertility, neurodegenerative, inflammatory and skin diseases. More recently, at the World Tomato Congress in 2006 scientists from Japan described the role of tomato lycopene in the prevention of emphysema and asthma in that country.

While many great advances have been made over the past decade, several key areas remain to be explored. These include:

1. Epidemiological studies to investigate the relationship between the consumption of tomatoes, tomato products and other sources of lycopene and cancer, cardiovascular diseases, osteoporosis, hypertension and neurodegenerative diseases.

2. Characterization of lycopene and its isomers with regard to their absorption, metabolism and biological activity.

3. Studies of the interactive relationships between lycopene and other carotenoids and dietary components in terms of the biological activity of lycopene.

4. Studies to investigate the underlying mechanisms of action of lycopene, apart from its antioxidant effects.

5. Clinical studies using well defined subject populations and disease end-points to investigate the role of tomato lycopene in the prevention and treatment of chronic diseases and to establish an optimal intake.

6. Obtaining more precise values for lycopene intake in different countries.

7. Research to develop tomato varieties with a high lycopene content that can be grown in high yield as well as being disease and pest-resistant.

8. Development of innovative nutraceutical and functional food products incorporating lycopene that are stable, bioavailable and flavorful.

9. Development of new process technology aimed at stabilizing lycopene and increasing its bioavailability.

10. Development of effective communication tools to educate health professionals and consumers about the health benefits of tomatoes and tomato products containing lycopene.

11. Development of methods to integrate international research collaborations and industrial activities to produce a cost effective system while maintaining scientific excellence.

12. Development of a comprehensive lycopene database that could be shared by researchers, health professionals, industrial participants, regulatory agencies and consumers.

13. Studies to investigate the beneficial interactions between lycopene and pharmaceutical drugs being used to treat chronic diseases.

14. Expanding the scope of the effects of lycopene beyond disease prevention to the actual treatment of chronic diseases such as cancer and cardiovascular disease.

NON-SCIENTIFIC GLOSSARY :

In simple terms, the best metaphor for describing what some of the terms contained in this volume mean is to describe the human body as a car. With a car, whatever the model, the same physical rules apply. The car will age with the passing of time and during this time it will be continuously attacked by exposure to the elements.

Oxidative Stress: Quite simply we can describe oxidative stress (oxidation) as the rusting of the the car. The metal reacts with oxygen forming a brown coloured oxide which ruins the paint work and what you are left with is rust. Now if you allow that to continue it won t be long before the continuous rusting action leaves an unsightly hole in the bodywork and its time for a new door panel and a re-spray. In human terms though we cannot simply go the body shop, we have to consider some other way to control the rusting action.

Antioxidants: Anti-rust treatment for your body. There are many nutritional elements which can do this but lycopene is one of the most effective. Tomatoes, especially processed tomato products also contain other nutrients which act and work together to increase their anti-rusting effects.

Phytochemicals: This group of chemicals are the plant s own self defence system against the sun and the elements. They are extremely potent and very effective and they also work for humans. Humans cannot make these chemicals in the body, they have to be ingested (eaten) as part of your healthy diet.

Carotenoids: Essentially, the color pigmentation of food as provided by Mother Nature. Lycopene is part of this family. Beta- carotene is what makes carrots orange and lycopene is what makes tomatoes red. Carotenoids are efficient free radical scavengers making them good for plants and good for us.

Free Radicals: These include oxy-radicals (or by another alias, singlet oxygen) and also ROS or reactive oxygen species. But not all free radicals are ROS and not all ROS are free radicals. It is these reactive molecules which cause the rusting action (oxidative stress). Free radicals effectively run around just looking for something to react with. That can be bad news if initiation, promotion or progress of a chronic disease is provoked. Antioxidants in the diet will find and quench (neutralize) these damaging molecules preventing further or ongoing harm. They can be stopped and the easiest way is by including more antioxidant rich foods in your diet.

Bioavailability: So how do we get the best from our dietary intake of foods which contain these chemicals? In the case of tomatoes, the heat from processing (effectively cooking) breaks open the cell matrix unlocking the most effective parts of the lycopene. This means you can absorb more of the right nutrients and enjoy an increased level of benefit to your health. This is bioavailability. Note, the same essential nutrients are found in fresh tomato but are much more available from processed. Therefore tomato juice or a good rich tomato pasta sauce provide some of the best ways to access these nutrients.

Industrial Perspective

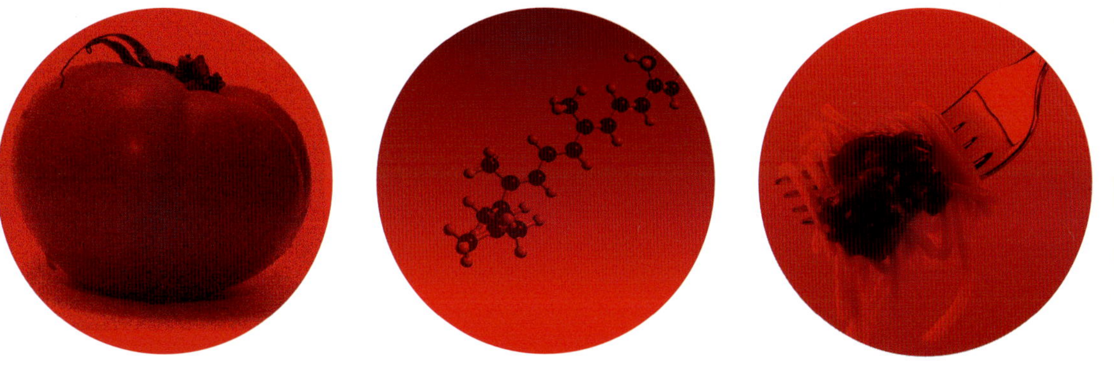

TOMATO LYCOPENE: INDUSTRIAL PERSPECTIVE

Dr. Zohar Nir
Dr. Dov Hartel
Lycored Natural Products Industries
Beer-Sheva, Israel

Introduction

The popularity of the tomato is based on its taste, color and the versatile role it plays in cooking. Since its introduction to the food industry, about 150 years ago, the tomato has become a major industrial crop with its popularity in cuisine spreading all over the world.

Tomato production in the USA and in Europe began to soar at the beginning of the 19th century with the advent of mass canning based on the introduction of juice extractors, efficient evaporators and new, high solids cultivars. Industrial tomato products are an integral part of the diet of people all around the world. Italian cooking, for example, has become synonymous with tomato sauce. Could one imagine pizza without tomatoes? Where would Mexican restaurants be without salsa? Potato chips without ketchup or a bloody Mary without tomato juice?

Tomato Lycopene and Health

Based on research findings scientists believe that tomatoes contribute more than culinary advantages. Series of studies conducted in leading research institutes indicate that diet rich in tomatoes decreases the occurrence of degenerative diseases such as various types of cancer and arteriosclerosis (1). Epidemiological studies combined with recent clinical trials have pushed tomatoes and tomato products from the culinary to the healthcare arena. Scientists are increasingly exploring the benefits of tomato phytonutrients as both preventative and adjunctive therapeutic agents, complementing established treatment protocol.

Dr. Edward Giovannucci, of the Department of Medicine of the Brigham and Women's Hospital and Harvard Medical School, reviewed 72 epidemiological studies looking at the role of tomatoes, tomato based products and blood lycopene level in reducing the risk of a variety of cancers. Dr. Giovannucci's review found that 57 of the 72 studies showed an inverse relationship between blood lycopene level (or tomato consumption) and cancer risk at a defined anatomical site. The evidence of the benefit of tomatoes was strongest for cancers of the prostate, lung and stomach (2).

Though much of the epidemiological work on lycopene has looked at its effect on cancer, there is growing evidence that lycopene is protective in several chronic diseases including cardiovascular disease (3) and age-related macular degeneration (4), as well as in the protection of the skin from erythema due to UV radiation (5). Initially, these findings were related to the high content of lycopene in tomatoes. However, closer scrutiny of the studies shows that that they were conducted with tomatoes, tomato products or with natural tomato extract and not with pure lycopene. Further investigations led scientists to believe that synergism between lycopene and other tomato phytonutrients enhances its ability to curb degenerative diseases.

Synergy

This synergistic effect of the natural composition of tomato phytonutrients was demonstrated in several studies including clinical research by Dr. Omer Kucuk with prostate cancer patients (6); a blind, placebo-controlled study by Esther Paran, MD, evaluating the effect of a tomato extract (oleoresin)(Lyc-o-Mato®), a standardized natural lycopene complex on 35 mildly hypertensive patients(7) ; Dr. Aviram's group research on the effects of tomato extract on LDL cholesterol (8,9); and the work done by Drs. Sharoni and Levi that demonstrated the effective synergy of tomato phytonutrients in reducing proliferation of prostate and breast cancer cells (10). This last work quite effectively showed that lycopene is not therapeutically effective when present at the relatively low levels normally found in the blood even after supplementation.

Tomato Lycopene

Effectiveness at the low lycopene concentrations that are possible to attain, occurs only when the lycopene is consumed along with other phytonutrients naturally present in the tomato. Thus the term "tomato lycopene" should refer to the natural mixture of lycopene, phytofluene, phytoene, beta carotene, tocopherols, etc. and not to lycopene alone.

However most of the publications use the term "lycopene" although they refer to results of studies that were conducted with the natural synergistic mixture as it exists in the ripe tomato. The health authorities are aware of the beneficial effect that tomato lycopene has on human health and look favorably on its consumption. It is an approved food color in Europe (E-160d), Japan and other countries. In the USA the FDA considers tomato lycopene as GRAS, has recently granted a CAP (color additive petition) for its use in food products and has given a partial qualified health claim stating that tomato lycopene may contribute to the prevention of prostate cancer. (Further scientific evidence will be required to fully satisfy the FDA in the United States although no such health claim qualification currently exists in Europe).

Tomato Lycopene in Human Diet

Although lycopene is present in several fruits (watermelon, red grapefruit, guava etc), tomatoes and tomato products account for more than 85% of lycopene intake in the human diet (11). People consume tomatoes in processed products, as fresh fruit in salads and in a variety of dishes. The consumption of tomatoes and of tomato products fluctuates widely according to location, season, availability and culinary preferences. The intake is high in countries where tomatoes are cultivated and processed. Thus the tomato is an essential component of the Mediterranean diet (scientists believe it to be one of the reasons this diet has a beneficial effect on health) and is consumed in large quantities in the countries which surround the Mediterranean sea; tomato consumption is also high in the USA and lower in Northern Europe. Currently there is no recommended daily allowance (RDA) for lycopene, although scientists who have conducted extensive research on the subject recommend a daily intake of between 5 and 10mg. This amount is present in one medium-size tomato, in half a glass of tomato juice or in less than one serving of tomato paste.

Bioavailability of Lycopene

Bioavailability is another important factor that has to be taken into consideration when lycopene intake is being investigated. Lycopene in the fresh tomato is locked in chromoplasts and protected by the cellular structure. This natural protection lowers the bioavailability. Processing denatures proteins, breaks down the cell walls and facilitates the release of lycopene from the chromoplast matrix, improving the digestion and bioavailability.

This explains the research findings that lycopene in processed tomato products is more bioavailable than in fresh tomato(12). Lycopene is insoluble in water but is soluble to some extent in oil. Therefore, as is the case with oil-soluble vitamins, the bioavailability of lycopene improves when it is consumed in the presence of lipids.

The effect of tomato lycopene research on the tomato industry

The results of tomato lycopene studies have been published in scientific journals and quoted in the news and wider media. As a result lycopene has become a household term. The general public is now much more aware of its beneficial effect on health and its contribution to the prevention of disease, though much work still needs to be done in keeping consumers informed of ongoing scientific discovery and verification of recent research results. Thus, the market is ready for tomato lycopene. The first products on the market that declared their lycopene content were food supplements. Functional foods soon followed and already there are food products on the supermarket shelves that are enriched with tomato lycopene and conventional tomato products that indicate lycopene content on their packaging and labels. This trend is surely going to spread since it is supported by a broad range of research results that indicate the beneficial effect of tomato lycopene on human health. The consumer wants to include lycopene in their diet and the best way to supply it is through the consumption of processed tomato products.

Conventional tomato products naturally contain lycopene and it seems a good business approach, instead of selling them as low price commodities, to present them as functional foods that contribute the desired lycopene to our diet. At present there are certain parameters that define the quality of a tomato product and currently they do not include lycopene content. It is thought that in the near future in addition to viscosity, total soluble solids and Hunter color parameters, tomato paste will be judged by its lycopene content. However, in order to achieve this the tomato industry will have to learn how to increase and standardize lycopene content in its products. Many efforts are currently underway across various sectors of the tomato industry to do precisely this in an endeavor to develop value added products which the market is now ready to receive.

This change consists of several integrated steps:

1. Use tomatoes with high lycopene content.

New lycopene rich tomato varieties (LRT) have recently been developed in a number of countries. In the development of LRT varieties only conventional breeding methods have been employed. Genetic manipulation has not involved in the process. In the breeding program, a combination of naturally occurring mutant pigment genes are introduced into parent lines carrying favorable traits required in good quality industrial tomatoes. Thus, LRT varieties, in addition to outstanding lycopene content, also give high and concentrated yield, have good solid and acid content as well as the typical tomato flavor. They have good color distribution throughout the fruit and are joint-less with good detachment of fruit. The LRT plant has proper habitus and good resistance to diseases and stress.

Since the LRT varieties contain twice as much lycopene as regular industrial tomatoes, by switching to the LRT tomatoes and without making any additional changes it is possible to double the lycopene content in conventional tomato products.
Lycopene content in tomatoes increases as the fruit matures. For highest lycopene content, ripe tomatoes should be used.

2. Prevent lycopene losses in processing.
Lycopene is naturally protected in the tomato tissue. Cutting, shredding, chopping and pulping increases exposure to oxygen and makes it vulnerable to degradation. Lycopene losses increase with longer processing time, higher temperatures and agitation. Takeoka *et al* (13) estimate that lycopene losses in tomato paste processing amount up to 28%.
At present, protection of lycopene from deterioration is not observed by the industry. This attitude will have to change due to the newly acquired importance of this carotenoid and the industry will have to introduce changes in their technology in order to assure a higher recovery of lycopene in tomato products.

3. Fortify and standardize tomato products with natural tomato lycopene.
Producers of natural tomato lycopene have developed and recently introduced into the market several proprietary products that can be used to increase and to standardize the content of lycopene in tomato products.
These are:

- Lycopene Rich Tomato Concentrate (LRTC) – Tomato concentrate with more than twice as much lycopene as in regular tomato paste.
- Spray dried lycopene rich fine tomato pulp.
- Aseptically packed lycopene rich tomato pulp.
- Tomato lycopene formulations in liquid and powder form, specially designed for various applications.

It is strongly believed that in the near future the scientific evidence that indicates the beneficial effect of tomato lycopene on health will dramatically and beneficially change the character of the tomato industry. In addition to their culinary advantages, tomato products will be judged according to their lycopene content.

REFERENCES:

1. Nguyen ML, Schwartz SI, Lycopene: Chemical and biological properties, Food Technology, 1999, 53 (2), 38-42.
2. Giovannucci E, Tomatoes, tomato-based products, lycopene, and cancer: Review of epidemiologic literature, Journal of the National Cancer Institute, Vol. 91, No. 4, Feb 17, 1999
3. Gomez-Aracena J, Sloots J, Garcia-Rodriguez A, et al, Antioxidants in adipose tissue and myocardial infarction in a Mediterranean area. The EURAMIC study in Malaga, Nutrition Metabolism and Cardiovascular Disease, 7376-82, 1997
4. Mares-Perlman JA, Brady WE, Klein BEK, Klein R, Bowen P, et al, Serum antioxidants and age-related macular degeneration in a population-based case control study, Archives of Ophthalmology, 1995; 113:1518-1523
5. Stahl W, Heinrich U, Wiseman S, Eichler O, Sies H, and Tronnier H, Dietary tomato paste protects against ultraviolet light-induced erythema in humans. Journal of Nutrition, 131:1449-51, 2001
6. Kucuk, O, Phase II Randomized Clinical Trial of Lycopene Supplementation before Radical Prostatectomy, Cancer Epidemiology Biomarkers and Prevention, August 2001
7. Engelhard Y, Paran E, The Anti-hypertensive Effect of Natural Antioxidants from Tomato Extract in Grade 1 Hypertensive patients, American Journal of Hypertension, May 2001
8. Fuhrman B, Ben-Yaish L, Attias J, Hayek T, Aviram M, Tomato's lycopene and -carotene inhibit low density lipoprotein oxidation and this effect depends on the lipoprotein vitamin E content, Nutrition, Metabolism and Cardiovascular Disease, 7:433-443, 1997
9. Fuhrman B, Volkova N, Rosenblat M, Aviram M, Lycopene Synergistically Inhibits LDL Oxidation in Combination with Vitamin E, Glabridin, Rosmarinic acid, Carnosic acid, or Garlic, Antioxidant Redox. Signaling (ARS) 2: 491-506, 2000
10. Levy Y, Sharoni J, Proceedings of the American Academy for Cancer Research, October 2002
11. Clydestale F.M. Lycopene: Critical Reviews in Food Science and Nutrition Vol. 39, Issue 3 1999
12. Giovannucci E, Ascherio A, Rimm E. B, Stampfer M. J, Colditz G. A, Willet W.C, Intake of Carotenoids and Retinol in Relation to Risk of Prostate Cancer . J Natl Cancer Inst 87: 1767-1776, 1995
13. Takeoka G.R.,Dao L,Flessa S, Gillespie D.M. , Jewell W.T. , Huebner B. , Bertow D. , Ebeler S. E., Processing Effects on Lycopene Content and Antioxidant Activity of Tomatoes Journal of Agricultural & Food Chemistry 49 (8): 3713-3717,Aug. 2001

Chemoprevention

Debra L. Bemis, Ph.D.
Director of Basic Science Research
Center for Holistic Urology
Columbia University Medical Center, New York.

As the Director of Basic Science Research for the Center of Holistic Urology at Columbia University Medical Center in New York, I have a deep interest in the potential chemopreventive actions of natural substances. Chemoprevention has been defined as the pharmacological intervention with naturally occurring or synthetic agents to prevent, arrest or reverse carcinogenesis.

What I find so compelling about this definition is the recognition of naturally occurring agents before synthetics. I believe this becomes a very empowering concept for cancer patients or anyone at risk as it suggests that there are ways for all of us to take action against this indiscriminating and unforgiving disease. One extremely accessible way is through diet.

In fact, it has been estimated that the adoption of a healthy diet could reduce the occurrence of colorectal, breast and prostate cancer by 66-75%, 33-55% and 10-20%, respectively. As highlighted in this book, a growing body of evidence is suggesting that the tomato is one dietary component that may have significant chemopreventive potential.

Compelling laboratory data demonstrate the ability of phytochemicals, found in tomatoes to inhibit cancer cell growth, and epidemiological studies have indicated that diets rich in tomato could lower the risk of developing prostate cancer. While research efforts must continue to define the health benefits of the tomato, projects such as this book allow us all to have access to important information and make active choices to adopt "chemopreventive" lifestyles.

Additional comment.I.

Britt Burton-Freeman, Ph.D., M.S.
University of California, Davis
Department of Nutrition

This text, "Tomatoes, Lycopene & Human Health, Preventing Chronic Diseases" contains an impressive quantity of relevant information for human health. The information communicated in this book provides insight to the important role processed tomatoes, lycopene and other lycopene-rich foods may play in promoting health and reducing disease risk world-wide. This book will be a valuable resource for consumers and professionals interested in diet and health.

Report to the General Assembly of AMITOM Tomato and Health Commission.

Juanjo Amézaga
President of the Tomato and Health Commission
AMITOM

As all of you know this commission has been dealing with the findings of new health scientific evidence about our tomato products and trying to disseminate the information not only to our members but also to specialised media and to the scientific community and political authorities.

The role of this commission was clearly established when the WPTC was created back in Pamplona 1998. The task was enormous due to the slow pace imposed by the scientific community. We did not want to spread non scientific evidence as the reputation of both AMITOM and the WPTC would have quickly fallen apart.

It s about time we all do something about this. We have to look at it as a long term approach, with long term returns. This is not a way of getting rid of stocks or selling at a higher price. It s a way of increasing and growing the market to provide our customers with better foods and to give replies to the public and political uproar caused by epidemic obesity and malnutrition.

Our politicians will support this approach as it gives them solutions. Our Health authorities are desperate to find ways to reduce the bill on healthcare related costs. Our consumers are also asking for an honest scientific approach and a clear message with truth and scientific evidence. Finally, with this book and publicly funded initiatives such as Lycocard, the answers are close at hand.

Additional comment.II.

Diane M. Barrett, PhD
Fruit & Vegetable Products Specialist
Dept. of Food Science & Technology
114 Food Science & Technology Building
University of California - Davis

Tomatoes are rich sources of macro nutrients such as Vitamin C, B and E, also fiber and additional compounds which we are still investigating such as lycopene, beta and alpha-carotene and polyphenolics. There are a multitude of additional compounds naturally found in tomatoes that may act as cofactors, or contributors to health.
We may have only scratched the surface in our understanding of nutritive components in tomatoes. Additionally, the use of supplements which contain only pure extractions of any one particular nutrient may miss some of the health benefits of whole tomato products. For this reason, I always advise consumers to eat whole tomatoes and their products.

Consumer Health Education

Gwen Young
Science Officer,
President of the Tomato and Health Commission
WPTC (World Processing Tomato Council)

As the chair for the Commission on Tomatoes and Health for the WPTC, I wanted to challenge the post to expand beyond the gathering of tomato and health data for WPTC membership and find a way to concisely share this information with the world. I passionately believe that people beyond the health conscious want to know just how healthy tomatoes are, but do not have the time nor the tools to conduct such research.

Fortuitously, through contacts with the scientific community, I began working with a fabulously driven publisher and well-versed teammate on the tomato and health quest. This book is the manifest tireless effort and at times feverishly impassioned work of numerous hours (months, years) by many volunteers to the delight and health reward of all. Increasing consumption of tomato-containing dishes offers absolute relevance to human health and nutrition globally.

With obesity and type II diabetes growing at epidemic rates, addressing healthy diets as part of a healthy lifestyle is paramount to the future of all people. Tomatoes and tomato products are known to some for their health and expected health benefits. But the average person is not aware of the vast quantity and quality of research that has been done in this area.

Thus, this book is the single most important educational platform from which to springboard mass education on the vast health benefits of tomatoes. Additionally, this book is a tool to gain support for further research to expand our understanding of the mechanisms of tomatoes and the full extent of the range of direct benefits to human health. It is essential therefore to continuously develop responsible and accurate health education strategies for consumers, the health professional sector, relevant political agencies and the food industry overall.

The Commission on Tomato & Health is charged with very important aims that were specifically placed during the foundation of the WPTC. These aims include:

- to collate information on the health benefits of tomato products
- to determine how the health arguments can be used to promote the consumption of tomato products

During my two year tenure heading up this commission these aims have been progressed by the following actions

- Assurance that WPTC endorsement is synonymous only with information that is accurate and scientifically credible.
- Through constant consultation with an independent scientific advisory board, transforming the WPTC website into an approved source of authority-based

information on tomatoes and health, for members, consumers, health professionals, advocacy groups and political agencies.

- Continuously expanding the information archives to include all current information on health claims and/or other government programs with the potential for increasing tomato product consumption / sales.
- Reinforcing the message that there is always a link between tomatoes as a part of a healthy diet and lifestyle in all that WPTC endorses.
- By completing the Global Tomato & Health Claim Review and Tomato Product Label Summary, presented in Parma (Oct 2005), OPVG & CLFP (both in Jan 2006).
- WPTC Supporting the scientific reference text: *Tomatoes, Lycopene & Human Health, Preventing Chronic Diseases",* Caledonian Science Press, Ltd.
- Formation of WPTC Fund for bulk purchase of this title and to support the distribution and promotion of tomato and health information, globally.

We are at an opportune moment in the tomato world, whereby through the actions of the WPTC we have been able to accomplish the previously impossible. A combination of global membership, cooperation and collaboration has resulted in the collation, endorsment, and publication of this text which brings the aims of the Commission on Tomato & Health to the heart of the WPTC. Here we have the most up to date overview of the key tomato and health research in a beautifully organized and accessible text; in every chapter the scientific research is complimented with plain language summaries.

Utilizing independent, scientific research will enable us to educate consumers on the special health benefits of tomato products. This is exactly the type of information doctors, consumers and political agencies have been waiting for. With obesity and chronic disease rates on the rise, it is time for a change of habits in food consumption and food culture. Including tomato products in the diet offers a way for all of us to eat healthily, enjoy good nutritious food and achieve whole body wellness. With such a delicious and versatile ingredient, what more enjoyable way could there be to protect your health?